The Circle of Fire

The Circle of Fire

The Metaphysics of Yoga

P. J. Mazumdar

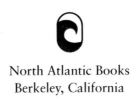

North Atlantic Books
Berkeley, California

Published by
North Atlantic Books
P.O. Box 12327
Berkeley, California 94712

Cover photo © iStockphoto.com/Devon Stephens
Cover and book design by Brad Greene
Printed in the United States of America

The Circle of Fire: The Metaphysics of Yoga is sponsored by the Society for the Study of Native Arts and Sciences, a nonprofit educational corporation whose goals are to develop an educational and cross-cultural perspective linking various scientific, social, and artistic fields; to nurture a holistic view of arts, sciences, humanities, and healing; and to publish and distribute literature on the relationship of mind, body, and nature.

North Atlantic Books' publications are available through most bookstores. For further information, call 800-733-3000 or visit our website at www.northatlanticbooks.com.

Library of Congress Cataloging-in-Publication Data

Mazumdar, Palash, 1970-
    The circle of fire : the metaphysics of yoga / Palash Mazumdar.
        p. cm.
    Summary: "Examines the Indian philosophy of advaita (non-dualism) in the light of theories and discoveries in the natural, physical, and medical sciences from ancient to modern times, and argues that advaita and the related practice of yoga provide the most suitable spiritual paths for the contemporary rational mind"—Provided by publisher.
    ISBN-13: 978-1-55643-670-3
    ISBN-10: 1-55643-670-X
    1. Advaita. 2. Yoga. 3. Philosophy and science. I. Title.
    B132.A3M385 2008
    181'.482—dc22
                                                                    2007049523

2 3 4 5 6 7 8 9 IBT 14 13 12 11 10

To my father,
the late Sri Ratneswar Mazumdar

∾

Acknowledgments

First, I would like to record my homage to the great teachers of the nineteenth century, Ramakrishna Paramahamsa and his disciple, Swami Vivekananda. This book is a tribute to their teachings and an enunciation of the philosophy that I understood most clearly from their writings and teachings.

My thanks also to my publishers, North Atlantic Books, and Richard Grossinger, who first gave me hope that my book could be published. A very special thanks to my editor, Hisae Matsuda, whose efforts were most critical in ensuring that the book eventually got published.

I would also like to record my gratitude to the Vivekananda Kendra in Guwahati, where I first made my contact with Indian philosophy and Yoga, and through whom I also acquired excellent books published by the Advaita Ashrama containing the deepest philosophical compositions of ancient India.

I would like to pay my deep respects to my father, the late Sri Ratneswar Mazumdar, whose simple but inspiring philosophy and hard work have always acted as a guide for me. My gratitude also to my mother, Usha Mazumdar, for her deep religious faith and spirituality which inspired and encouraged me. Also, special thanks to my sisters for all the animated discussions we shared around meals on so many diverse topics, which have always been so intellectually stimulating.

And lastly, a final thanks to my wife Nita for her helpful and patient support during the long process of publication.

Contents

Part One
Jnanakanda: Knowledge

Introduction: The Origins of Life, the Universe, and Indian Thought

Then who knows from whence came this existence?
From whence came this universe?
He, the foremost in all this creation,
Who is controlling it all from the highest of the Heavens—
Perhaps He knows, or perhaps even He knows not!

—Rig Veda X.129

T he mystery of our existence has tantalized us through the ages. The need to understand our place in the universe and the reason why everything happens as it does has spurred the best minds in all civilizations. Trying to pierce through this uncertainty, most seers faced the same problems and came up with broadly the same answers, although the paths they took to obtain those answers were quite different.

When we look at the main existential questions, we are at once faced with a number of paradoxes that seem impossible for our minds to reason out. In considering space and time, for example, we come across one such contradiction. We cannot conceive of the world being finite in space, for immediately the question of what then lies beyond this limit presents itself. Nor can we hold in our minds the concept that the universe is infinitely large and never has an end no matter how far we travel in it. Similarly, we cannot conceive of a beginning or end of time, nor can we conceive of ages which do not have a beginning in the past or an end in the future.

But yet we know that both time and space must be either finite or infinite, as we cannot conceive of anything being both finite and infinite either. Our minds, it seems, just do not have enough brainpower to solve this riddle.

We have not been able to make much sense of life either. Is life just the sum total of all the reactions going on in a living body, or is it something much bigger than that? What, then, is a living body? We have no hesitation in calling an amoeba a living body, but within our own bodies there are also billions of cells, which are as "living" as an amoeba. Is our own "life" something larger than the lives of these, our constituent living units? At what stage can we separate our own "life" from the lives of our cells, such as our brain cells?

Although trying to define life presents such problems, we cannot deny life either. How did life originate? We laugh now at the old belief in spontaneous generation, where scorpions are born from cow dung or worms from rotten food. But in fact our present theory of life also holds that life can and did originate from nonlife, only we push it back millions of years and say it happened only once.

We have not been able to understand our own identity either. What really is this "I"? It certainly is not just our body, for we can cut off one arm and still remain the same person. Also, turning our minds inward, trying to separate out our own ego is an impossible task. It is difficult to grasp that our entire identity is confined to this particular body only, and can never traverse beyond the body. It seems intuitive to us that our self, our "I" is a separate being, who performs all actions like thinking, sensing, moving, and so on. Yet when we look inwards, we cannot make the distinction between our thoughts and the person who is doing the thinking. At the same time, we also cannot accept that there is no separate "I," that it is just a stream of thoughts, emotions, and sensations that make up our identity.

The world presents vast areas where the mind has to turn back for want of light. This confusion gives rise to the idea of something beyond the world to explain it: the concept of God. Only such a supernatural power seems to explain all that we see around us. Every culture eventually arrives at this concept of God as a lid on the disorder.

However, there has been a dramatic advancement in our knowledge in the last two hundred years. Several of the great mysteries that frustrated mankind in previous ages have been solved. We now know far more of life and far more of the universe than we ever have in all of history. The need for God as an explanation has considerably lessened as we found satisfactory answers that do not need an outside cause. A radical departure from our previous ideas of God and religion would be needed to reconcile them with the growth in scientific knowledge in the past two centuries. The advances that have proved to be the most challenging for our old philosophical concepts have been in the life sciences, physics, and the medical sciences.

I

The Natural Sciences

A thousand heads had primal Man,
A thousand eyes, a thousand feet:
Encompassing the earth on every side,
He exceeded it by ten fingers' breadth.
That Man is this whole universe,
What was and what is yet to be,
The Lord of immortality.

    —Rig Veda VII.76

The origination of life and the diversity of living things have been some of the strongest arguments for the existence of God. In the past, the unfathomable beauty of life had no easy answers, and only a divine conception seemed equal to its mystery. Nothing else could explain how life came into existence and why mankind was so obviously superior to all other life forms.

Positing God as a supreme creator solves this vital question. Life then becomes a sacred gift, something that by definition is beyond human comprehension. Also, an important implication is that God created the human race to be superior to other creatures. The world then becomes a testing ground in which humans are placed to fulfill a divine purpose. Much of religion consists of an interpretation of what this divine purpose is and what it means in our lives.

The idea that changed virtually all our thinking about how the human race came to exist was the theory of evolution, propounded mainly by Charles Darwin in the middle of the nineteenth century. The notion that life was not created suddenly but rather evolved gradually from other forms was not a new idea and had been held by philosophers since ancient times. This was the theory of the most ancient of the Hindu philosophies, the *Samkhya* school. But unlike Darwin's practical ideas of the evolution of species, Samkhya theory involved specific principles of nature, which arose from more general forms, and in turn gave rise to more specific forms and so on until the development of mankind. It was an idea of evolution based on imaginary principles and entities.

However, Darwin was to give a far more practical and scientific theory. He showed that the diversity of the different life forms in the world did not need a creator but could be easily explained by simple laws of nature. Nature did not have a purpose but merely followed a course determined by the odds. He demonstrated that the higher forms of life were developed from the lower ones. This led to the inevitable conclusion that man, too, was not created, but merely developed from other life forms. Darwin and other scientists soon had irrefutable proof in the form of fossils and biological studies, which proved their theory beyond reasonable doubt, although the finer details may still be debated.

As could be expected, this theory unnerved all traditional religions, and there were vehement protests against it by the reigning high priests. It shook the thinking of all persons; from a vague belief that humans were indeed superior and had a special place in the sun, they had now to believe that they were merely one in a chain of circumstances, with all kinds of slimy creatures and monkeys as ancestors.

The psychological blow to the people of that age must have been immense. We now faced a world where we were still at the top of the pyramid, but we were also very much an inseparable part of it. We stood at this position not because of any wise dispensation from above, but because we had fought and killed with the rest of them—and done it better. There was no fundamental gap, no place where God could have intervened to grant us a higher status. There was now no divine purpose behind our existence.

In addition to the fossil record, the evidence from the anatomy and chemistry of our bodies also shows our common origin with other "lower" life forms. For instance, genetic data has provided fresh proof, such as the almost identical genetic codes (ninety percent) between chimpanzees and humans. Various other studies of comparative physiology and anatomy demonstrate beautifully the different stages of evolution of our organs and functions, such as eyesight, urine formation, and so forth.

Of course most dualists, who accept unquestioningly the concept of a divine creator, do not accept evolution. Besides them, there are people who, while not being such orthodox dualists, still reject evolution. But most of this rejection is totally irrational and egotistical, being of the "What, me descended from monkeys?!" variety. To get around evolution, one recent idea proposed is that man originated in some way from travelers from outer space. According to this, the aliens mated with pre-humans (they must have been really desperate!) and gave rise to our race. In this way, a touch of the celestial is retained for our origin through these modern divine beings. This does not, however, solve the problem, as we still have to explain how the aliens evolved in the first place. Either *they* would have had to evolve from monkeys on their own planet, or we have to posit another super-alien race for them, and so on. There is really no getting away from our ancestors.

One of the strongest objections in rejecting evolution is that if we give up the idea of a creator behind the world, we will also be giving up a vital part of our life, the strength that the concept of an absolute being gives to us. There is no denying that the need for spirituality in our life is as important a part of our makeup as the need for intellectual, emotional, and physical satisfaction. The concept of evolution destroys the basic beliefs of most traditional religions, where it is either a case of accepting the religion or accepting evolution.

However, this is not true of all religions. Hinduism and Buddhism are the two most important religious traditions that can support us spiritually while at the same time allowing us to accept evolution and all other scientific knowledge as true. Understanding Advaitism (non-dual Hindu philosophy) and Buddhism gives us a concept of religion that provides us spiritual strength through the idea of a higher absolute, without forcing us to reject science and rationalism.

The seminal idea in evolution is that there is no fixed purpose or direction behind it. The two forces that drive evolution are sexual selection and selection for survival. Sexual selection favors organisms that are most attractive or powerful sexually, as these individuals mate more and hence have more offspring (for instance, birds with more colorful feathers or males with bigger horns). Selection for survival favors those individuals who have an extra something to survive in their environment, such as giraffes with longer necks to feed on higher leaves. Each animal fits into its own particular niche in the complex environment, and in turn changes the environment to a certain extent, perhaps creating new niches for other creatures or disturbing other creatures in their niches and driving them to extinction.

Sexual selection and selection for survival are not purposive forces that create evolution. They are simply terms used to describe certain processes. Nature does not have a mechanism to select for sexual advantage; it is only that those creatures that by mutation acquire a certain quality that lets them mate more automatically produce more offspring. Similarly, those that have qualities that enable them to survive in a difficult environment also automatically have more offspring. Evolution theory thus showed that there is no active principle, whether divine or in nature, that guides or propels evolution. This fundamental truth changed all our thinking on God and our own existence.

Another idea that developed parallel to the idea of evolution or the origin of different species is that of the origin of life itself. Evolution explained how different species developed, but it still did not explain how the very first life form originated. Through fossils, we can trace back the chain to the simplest sea creatures, but beyond a certain limit fossils are nonexistent, because the earliest life forms were too tiny and made of soft tissue. But Darwin's theory of higher forms of life originating from the lower already suggested that there must have been some simplest life forms from which all others originated.

The collapse of the belief in the divine origin of individual species led to the collapse of the belief in the divine origin of life, and more scientific ideas were developed. Darwin preferred not to go into this aspect, but by the middle of the nineteenth century it was being forcefully suggested with scientific backing that these simplest life forms could have originated from nonliving matter.

It is now known that the early atmosphere of the earth was

very different from today's, with an abundance of hydrogen rather than oxygen. Our present atmosphere adds oxygen to anything that comes into contact with it, as demonstrated by iron's transformation into rust (iron oxide); this is called an oxidizing chemical reaction. In contrast, the previous atmosphere added hydrogen; this is called a reducing chemical reaction. In such an atmosphere, organic molecules would be easily created. In an interesting experiment, which has been repeated, a soup containing the early atmosphere and gases of the primitive world were mixed together in the same proportions as must have existed at the earliest time. These were then subjected to heat and electrical discharges to duplicate the violent storms of the early world and allowed to "stew" for some time in these conditions. Then, surprisingly, it was found that after some time amino acids, the first building blocks, were created in the mixture. Amino acids have also been found in the most unlikely places, such as comets and asteroids, where they must have formed accidentally during the turbulent passages of these rocks.

It is not difficult from here to imagine these amino acids coalescing accidentally and then forming primitive proteins. Out of these, those that had the strongest bonds would have been the most stable. Those molecules, which had the capacity to absorb energy from the surrounding environment into them so that their bonding would be faster or stronger, would have become more plentiful. Thus gradually those pre-life forms with the greatest potential for life became the most plentiful. Any such line that accidentally acquired even the crudest form of self-replication—perhaps nothing more than the formation of a regular sequence of chemicals with a tendency to break off at fixed intervals—would have proliferated, and, because of its reproductive capacity, could be termed the first life. Eventually these early forms gave rise to the whole course of evolution leading up to us.

The concepts of evolution and the origin of life left no role for God to intervene at any stage. Life is transmitted in an unbroken chain, and this chain has been continuous since the first dawn of life. The earliest life forms, the prokaryotes, are virtually immortal. There is no inevitable death for them unless they are killed accidentally. During multiplication they simply split into two daughter cells so that, in a sense, the first such organisms still continue to exist. An amoeba of today can be said to be the same organism living from the beginnings of life on earth.

Even in higher creatures such as humans there is no beginning of life, as the egg and sperm of the parents are already living. When these unite to form a new organism, there is no sudden grant of life but only a continuation of the lives of the egg and the sperm, which in turn are a continuation of the lives of the parents. There is no point where God has to step in and grant life to a nonliving organism, either in the course of any individual life or in the whole history of life. This eliminates the most important role of God in all traditions.

Another important revelation, especially in recent decades, was in the study of our natural environment and wildlife. Nature was long considered to be just another resource to be exploited. The unraveling of its immense complexity has been quite humbling. Darwin had already suggested that our physical and psychological characteristics are also evolved from other animals. This theory has been not just vindicated but greatly enlarged through our present knowledge of wildlife.

In everything that we do—in our activities, tastes, creativity, and so on—we can find a precedent in the animal kingdom. Our taste in sense objects matches quite closely to that of the animals. We may find beauty in flowers, but this beauty was meant to attract insects that apparently have the same sense of style. Similarly, we enjoy the scent of flowers and the taste of fruits, when in fact these are meant for insects and birds.

Even our higher tastes have their clear counterpart in the animal world. The musical notes of bird songs are as charming for us as the female birds for which they are meant. Our dancing has a clear precedent in the mating dance of birds. Birds are also known to arrange their nests in as artistic and creative a fashion as possible to attract their mates. Birds like the jackdaw seem to decorate their nests with brightly colored baubles gathered from the streets.

Even our so-called higher emotions are clearly mirrored in the animal world. Parental bonding prevails throughout the mammalian world. Other social bonds are clearly seen, especially in herding animals. Elephants are known to mourn for days near the body of one of their herd when it dies. Many birds mate for life, and some, like the Brahmini duck, will stand crying beside its mate if it is killed, until it also dies. It would be hard work trying to find such love in our own race. The importance of having a leader to make decisions and the discipline to follow the leader's directions is also clearly seen. The social bonds between herding animals are as complex and strong as in any human society. All this has led to the realization that we owe most of the fundamentals of human culture to our animal ancestors.

The progress of our knowledge in the origin and course of life poses a serious challenge to the traditional concept of religion. The dominance of God is derived in most religions from his importance in creating and sustaining life. But that role cannot be believed in any more. Science has shown that there is no need to posit any divine hand in the origin of life; the human race does not occupy a central position, nor was it created differently from the rest.

This new knowledge has demolished the beliefs at the core of most religions, and as a result much of their doctrines have become redundant. It is untenable now for religions with pre-evolutionary concepts to sustain their teachings in the light of this new knowledge. Only religions that can accept evolution and other scientific discoveries can achieve harmony with our intellectual progress and spiritual needs.

The Physical Sciences

There the sun does not shine, nor the moon and the stars; nor do these flashes of lightning shine. How can this fire? He shining, all these shine; through His luster all these are illumined.

—Katha Upanishad, II.ii.15

Through most of history, almost all models of the universe held that humans were at the heart of it all. It seemed common sense to assume that the sun and all the stars revolved around the earth, with the earth as the center of the cosmos. This fit perfectly with the belief that the whole of creation was a theater made solely for humanity, to please or to test us according to the prevailing theology. It is difficult to realize now how narrow this view of the universe was, but the knowledge that we take for granted today of the universe's vastness was something totally beyond the comprehension of most people until recently.

Some challenges to this idea of human supremacy were already present a long time ago, originating from a few astronomers and mathematicians. Aristarchus (320 BCE), a Greek astronomer, was the first to suggest that the earth and the planets revolved around the sun. Aryabhatta (600 CE), an Indian mathematician, not only proffered his view of the heliocentric world but even calculated the orbits of the planets and the sizes of the earth and the moon. The view that the stars were sun-like objects also seemed to have been known to Indian astronomers. But, by and large, there was very little scientific knowledge and inquiry into the cosmos. Although there were very accurate observations and calculations of the movements of the heavenly bodies, there was little knowledge of what these bodies actually were. In India the stars and planets were deified and were seen as mysterious objects ruled by various gods. As they reigned in heaven, they were believed to have power over human fate, and as such the study of astrology was the main motivation for all inquiry into the heavens. The vastness of the universe was totally unknown.

In the West, too, although the nature of these stars was not known, their movements were well-recorded. Complex models were proposed with the earth as the center of the universe, surrounded by revolving spheres in which the planets and stars were embedded. The stars were seen as jewels, which were embedded in these spheres. This was the Aristotelian model. To explain the path of planets, Ptolemy further modified the model, and his became the uniformly accepted model for the cosmos.

The march toward a better understanding of the universe came with Nicolaus Copernicus (1473–1543), who asserted the heliocentric position of the solar system and affirmed that the planets were bodies similar to the earth. But the real jump toward a scientific view of the cosmos came with Galileo Galilei (1564–1642). He not only accepted the Copernican theory, but backed it up with scientific data collected from his new telescopes. Galileo also discovered that the planets were different from the stars and had their own moons, which revolved around them.

Not surprisingly, this was a serious challenge to the prevailing creationist philosophies. It was strongly opposed by the church, which rose to the challenge, made Galileo recant everything, and then imprisoned him. But Galileo's theory was backed by solid evidence and would not be denied. Galileo had also introduced a new method of investigation into the world: the science of experimentation. The famous—perhaps apocryphal—story of how Galileo went to the tower of Pisa and dropped two objects to test Aristotle's theory that heavier objects would fall faster is an important turning point in human history. Before this, all knowledge was accumulated by thinking alone; this vast shift to adopt the methods of science ensured rapid gains in humanity's understanding of the world. With the irrefutable evidence gathered by observations, scientists gradually began to accept the heliocentric idea of the solar system, although it was still far from general acceptance.

The next scientist who helped change much of the thinking on the universe was Isaac Newton (1643–1727). Besides his other work on optics and mathematics, he discovered and laid out his theory of the universal law of gravitation. It had a profound impact on the thinking of the generation. The fact that every particle in the universe attracted every other particle with essentially the same proportional force indicated an absolute wholeness of creation. Everything from the atoms to the planets was related and followed the same laws. Newer and more advanced telescopes also gradually brought out another startling fact, that of the size and scale of the solar system. Newton also asserted that the stars were the same as our sun and the universe was a sea of stars.

So by the end of the eighteenth century, the narrow view of the universe was being broken down for a much wider outlook. But although several traditional views, such as an earth-centric universe, were broken down, the much larger and more complex universe that was now visualized still had a perfect consonance of creation. This unity pointed squarely to the presence of a creator, and thus creationist theories were further supported. There was total order and harmony in the universe, and it was logical to see a grand old Ruler who had created, and presided over, this harmony and order. This Creator had made the world in a certain way and given it certain laws, and the whole world followed these laws and worked itself out so that all His plans were fulfilled. The vastness of the universe and the puniness of humans in relation to it also made the Creator seem unlimited to mankind. Everything was related to everything else, and worked in a closed and symbiotic order. Thus, although orthodox Christian concepts were not strictly followed, the new understanding of the universe, both in philosophical and in scientific terms, supported the concept of a creator.

But by the beginning of the nineteenth century, this view of the universe began to come under serious challenge. The first challenge arose regarding the concept of the atom. The atom was earlier conceived as a tiny indestructible unit, which was God-given and out of which He created the entire known universe and caused it to follow His laws. But the atom under scientific investigation began to reveal its secrets. The work of scientists such as John Dalton (1766–1844) began to show that atoms were particles with mass and properties, which combined with each other to form molecules. The work of Dmitri Ivanovich Mendeleev (1834–1907) showed all properties of matter to be the properties of their atoms. Michael Faraday (1791–1867) had already begun to show that atoms were not all matter; they also had electrical charge. As more knowledge of the atom was gathered, it came to be seen as a functional entity that followed known laws. This made it difficult to see God's hand in its creation or function.

Finally, in 1897, the electron was discovered by George Paget Thomson and its mass was calculated. Thus atoms were shown not to be indestructible after all, but rather composed of smaller units, the subatomic particles. The concept of a single indivisible unit of the universe, the atom, had collapsed, and instead there was a multitude of fundamental building blocks. The structure of the universe, it turned out, was diverse instead of simple and harmonious, and it increased in complexity as our scientific knowledge grew. Also, at its most basic, there was certainly nothing from outside that guided the universe; it followed its own laws.

Even as the knowledge of the microscopic world was changing the old concepts, newer challenges came from the study of the macrocosm. At the end of the eighteenth century there was still no appreciation of the size of the universe. But from about two hundred years ago, astronomers were slowly beginning to understand its vastness. Until then, humanity's vision was confined to the solar system, with no knowledge of the distance of the stars. The first star was measured in 1838 by Friedrich Bessel. It is difficult now to realize the impact that the distance, which was about ten light years, must have had on the imagination of people of that period, who were rudely awakened to a completely different concept of the universe. Several other stars were measured after that. But it was only in the twentieth century that indirect methods of measuring star distance were discovered and Edwin Hubble measured the distance of other galaxies. The size of the known universe had now become unbearably vast and beyond human comprehension. It would be absurd now to think of humans as being central to the universe, lost as we are in this measureless space.

Another, even more serious challenge rose from trying to understand the laws that governed the stars. As there was greater progress in observing the motion of the stars, several discrepancies were noticed that did not seem to follow the old Newtonian laws. The nature of light, especially its speed, also began to attract greater attention. Various scientists analyzed the behavior of light in different ways, both as particles and as waves. This already contradicted previous theories. The Michelson-Morley experiment in 1897 showed that light speed was constant under all conditions. It was this experiment that led to the theory that changed all our concepts of the universe; the brilliant interpretation of this experiment's result led to Albert Einstein's special theory of relativity in 1905 and general theory of relativity in 1915.

The relativity theories effectively tore down the whole of the Newtonian conception of the universe. In Newton's world, everything had its time and place and followed fixed laws. But with the relativity theory, this surety of the world disappeared. Einstein related both time and space to the observer. Suddenly there was no absolute time or space, and, with this, the old idea of the universe as a harmonious whole was effaced. No object in the world has an absolute reality. If we consider, for example, the length of a body, then different observations of this length by observers in different frames will give differing figures. All these differing figures are equally true; we cannot consider any of them to be absolutely true and the others false. Hence no object in the universe has an absolute length; all figures for its length are only relatively true. This is also true for its breadth, mass, speed, and so forth.

Even as the theories of relativity were being framed, important challenges were being posed to it by more knowledge of the atom and subatomic particles. The advent of *quantum physics* began with Max Planck, who in 1900 introduced his quanta theory that energy is emitted in packets, thus giving a physical and quantifiable identity to energy. This was the final blow to the old Newtonian theories. Energy, along with such properties as charge, became a mathematical quantity that physicists used in their calculations along with traditional properties such as mass. All radiation was now said to have both a particle and a wave existence, which soon led to the concept that in fact all matter had both particle and wave characteristics. Along with Einstein's famous theorem, $E=MC^2$, matter and energy became interchangeable and part of a spectrum, at one end of which was matter, and at the other end, energy.

This merger now led to another very important discovery, Werner Heisenberg's Uncertainty Principle, which proposes that it is impossible to determine both the position and the velocity of a particle at the same time. What it effectively meant was that particles do not have a true existence in the sense that we understand—being both matter and energy simultaneously, which is contradictory to our natural experience—and that they also have several different states of existence. Newer discoveries in the field of submicroscopic particles continue to reveal very strange particles that show all manner of paradoxical behavior, such as appearing out of and vanishing into nothingness. Besides the laws of science, their behavior seems to defy our logic and rationality. Quantum physics now deals with a world where there is, apparently, almost total anarchy.

The theories of relativity and quantum physics tore down not just Newton's gravitational laws but the whole traditional idea of God. The lack of any absolute reality in the universe contradicts our entire view of creation. Quantum mechanics shows a world where the smallest particles do not have a distinct, fixed existence, but instead experience several states of existence simultaneously. Therefore, the interactions between particles do not follow a single path and have ambiguous results. There is thus no scope for a supreme power such as God to intervene and control the effects.

The fact that randomness is built into the world also presents a fundamental contradiction to the theory that God had decreed the laws initially and the world was working out according to His plans. It means that, no matter what laws had been given initially, the outcomes of each event would not work out in a fixed, pre-determined manner but could be any one of several outcomes. There was no way in which God or any power would be able to decree the shape or nature of the world by decreeing the initial positions and laws. The world had worked itself out in this way entirely by chance. Hence the real universe is now known to be far different from the commonsense view that comes naturally to us. The traditional concepts of God, which arose from such a view of the universe, cannot coexist with our modern-day physics.

The Medical Sciences

~ 3

*Man, O Gautama, is Fire. Of this, the open mouth is its fuel,
the vital force its smoke, speech its flame, the eye its embers,
and the ear its sparks.*

—Brihadaranyaka Upanishad, VI.ii.13

The human body has been a source of mystery since ancient times. Even today, the presence of life and consciousness in the body is impossible to explain in terms of matter alone. It was inconceivable that this flesh and blood alone could account for the presence of life. The other, equally great mystery about the body is its physical working. What makes the blood flow in our veins and food get absorbed into energy? How do the senses work? How, for example, do we see with our eyes? While the eye itself is clearly a material object, vision, it was felt, could not be explained in terms of matter alone. Thought also seemed something totally transcendent and non-material. It was felt that no solution in nature could account for all these wonders of our body. The only explanation seemed something extraordinary, something divine: the soul.

The soul is a fundamental concept of all religions and is as important as God, with as many different definitions. It denotes the presence of the spirit in the body, being something that resides in the body yet is not a part of it, "the ghost in the machine." It provides the religious explanation for the body's capacity to sustain life and consciousness.

The concept of the soul means that in essence we are not our bodies but something divine and transcendent. This gives religions justification for their existence, as each claims to offer our true identity, our soul, some kind of reward for following the religion's dictums—even when such teachings seem contrary to the demands of our bodies. It also means that we are, in principle, immortal, and the present life in our bodies is a mere shadow. The soul allows religions to promise rewards for all eternity in return for obedience in this life. The soul provides the *raison d'être* for all religious teaching.

But here too science has changed all our concepts. Modern medical knowledge has now deciphered many of the mysteries of the body, and its functioning is understood to a great extent, without any need to posit something outside the physical body to account for the presence of life. Our present knowledge has shown that the functioning of the human body is, in fact, a mechanical working-out of the laws of physics and biochemistry. A study of the origin, structure, and functions of the fundamental constituents of our body, the proteins, shows us how self-sufficient and systematic our bodies are.

Proteins form the bulk of the structure of human body, and they play the main part in all its physiological actions. Proteins are composed of long chains of molecules called amino acids. In the human body, proteins are composed of a total of twenty amino acids, such as lysine and glutamine, and different sequences of them constitute the different proteins. A virtually infinite variety of such chains of amino acids is possible, and this accounts for the very large number and variety of proteins found in biological life.

The main atom in an amino acid molecule, as in almost all other molecules in the human body, is the carbon atom.

Life on earth is based on the carbon atom, and all organic chemicals have carbon as their base. Carbon is so important because it has as many as six valences, or "arms," to which other atoms can be attached, and it is also very stable. Because of carbon's large number of potential links, like the central piece in a do-it-yourself toy, several atoms (up to six) can be attached to a single carbon atom on its arms, and when other carbon atoms are attached, very large and complex molecules can be created. Some other atoms, such as silicon, also have this property, so we may well find silicon-based life on some other planet.

In the case of amino acids, a central carbon atom combines with oxygen, hydrogen, and nitrogen atoms on its different arms to form an amino acid molecule. Different arrangements of the other atoms give different amino acids, each with slightly different properties. The final three-dimensional shape of a protein and its properties are determined by the amino acids forming the protein and the electrophysiological interactions between them. A change of even a single amino acid could change the shape of the whole protein and its properties.

The DNA in the chromosomes of our cells directs the formation of proteins. Like a protein, the DNA (deoxyribonucleic acid) molecule is composed of a long chain, in this case a chain of a chemical called a nucleotide. Each nucleotide unit has a nitrogenous base, to which is attached a pentose (meaning *containing five carbon atoms*) sugar group at one end and a phosphate group at the other. The sugar and phosphate groups of adjacent nucleotides link to one another, and the nitrogenous base projects out from the backbone of this chain. A chromosome, of which there are forty-six in each cell of our bodies, is composed of a multitude of such long DNA molecules loosely intertwined together.

There are four nitrogenous bases, named adenine (A), thymine (T), guanine (G), and cytosine (C), projecting out from the DNA molecule. The bases are thus arranged in a long sequence, such as A-C-T-C-G .... It is this sequence that carries all the information about us and determines our whole physical existence. Each triplet of bases codes for a specific amino acid, and the entire chain of code letters thus codes for a chain of amino acids and ultimately for a protein. Each such complete chain of letters in the DNA of our chromosomes that codes for an entire protein is called a gene. Thus, a gene is nothing but a code for a particular protein, which it creates in the body.

All the genetic information that a chromosome carries is only the information about the structure of our proteins. Proteins perform such a vital role that the slightest difference in this information causes the difference from one individual to another, and also the difference between species. A unit of the hormone insulin, for example, contains fifty-one amino acids and hence will have a chain of fifty-one triplets of bases coding for it. Pig insulin differs from the human only in having the amino acid alanine instead of threonine at one place out of the fifty-one, but this difference is significant enough to alter its effect in our bodies. Difference of genes between two individuals means nothing more than a difference of a few nitrogenous bases in the genes. This gives rise to slightly different proteins with different amino acids at a few places, which might give blue eyes to one person and black to another, or different rates of certain chemical reactions in the body, and so on.

The formation of proteins from these codes occurs in a mechanical assembly-line manner. The fundamental rule here is the base-pairing rule, by which an adenine base will pair only with a thymine base and vice versa, or A~T. In the same way, cytosine can pair only with guanine and vice versa, or C~G. A and T are therefore called complementary to each other, as are G and C. A chain in which all the As of the original are replaced by Ts, Ts by As, Gs by Cs, and Cs by Gs is called complementary to the original. Two DNA strands, complementary to each other, twist around themselves to form the complete DNA double helix of our chromosomes. Each chromosome carries vast numbers of such DNA molecules, along with their encoded genetic information.

DNA does not form proteins directly but through an intermediary template, the mRNA, or messenger RNA. RNA is very similar to DNA, except that the sugar group in RNA nucleotides is ribose instead of deoxyribose, and some other small differences.

A molecule called the RNA polymerase controls the formation of mRNA from DNA. RNA polymerase unwinds the DNA molecule and lays down a strand of RNA that contains the same sequence of complementary bases. In this way the code on the DNA is copied onto the RNA but in a complementary manner— that is, As for Ts, and so on. Thus, the entire code for a single protein, the gene contained in the DNA, is faithfully transcribed complementarily onto the RNA. This new RNA, containing the complementary image of the DNA gene, now gets separated and lies in the "pulp" of the cell, which is the part of the cell outside the nucleus. It is this mRNA that will actually form the protein. The sequence of bases on the mRNA molecule determines the sequence of amino acids in the protein that it will form. Each triplet of bases on the RNA now stands for a particular amino acid. AAA stands for lysine, GAA stands for glutamine, and so forth. Each triplet is called a codon, and the complete sequence of codons in the RNA, which stands for one protein, is called a *genetic code* (as opposed to a *gene*, which is contained in the DNA). This genetic code in the mRNA is, of course, a complementary copy of the gene in the original DNA in the chromosome.

The formation of proteins from mRNA is called translation. To do this, another component is needed: the tRNA, or transfer RNA. There are specific tRNAs for each of the twenty different amino acids, and these tRNAs—with their attached amino acids— are found free in the cell material, the pulp. Each tRNA molecule consists, on one end, of a loop that holds its particular amino acid. On the other end it contains a triplet of bases, the anticodon, which is complementary to the codon for that particular amino acid on the mRNA. For example, the tRNA for lysine would hold a molecule of lysine at one end, and at the other, the anticodon of AAA—that is, TTT. Thus, for lysine, the code on the gene on the DNA would be TTT, whereas on the codon in the mRNA it would be AAA, and TTT again on the tRNA.

When translation occurs, a cellular component called the ribosome moves over the mRNA strand and joins each codon in the mRNA to its specific anticodon tRNA molecule. The codon (on the mRNA) and anticodon (on the tRNA) fit into each other like a lock and its key. As the different tRNA molecules are lined up on the mRNA strand, the amino acids attached to them also get lined up in the correct order, so that there are three chains side by side: the mRNA on one side, the tRNA in the middle, and the amino acids on the other side. In this way, the correct sequence of amino acids—which was coded originally in the gene of the DNA—is finally formed. From the gene in the DNA, the sequence gets transferred to the genetic code in the mRNA, then to the proper sequence of tRNA, and then finally to the proper sequence of amino acids. The sequence of amino acids is then joined up, and the basic protein strand gets separated. The protein's basic structure—a long chain of amino acids—now assumes a complex three-dimensional shape that determines its actions and properties.

These proteins are the workhorses of the human body. They are by far the most important components in the body, as it is they that run the vast enterprise of keeping us 'alive.' They perform or help to run the vast array of physical, chemical, and electrical functions in the human body. There are a very large number of such proteins in our body, each with its own specific function. Because of their structure, proteins can have a virtually infinite variety of configurations, both in their physical shape and in their chemical components. Each amino acid has its own chemical properties, and the shape of the protein can present a cluster of amino acids at a particular end, which will then have a distinct chemical property suitable for a specialized function.

Each protein is really an extremely ingenious robot that performs its functions with the lowest energy expenditure possible. Evolution has produced a degree of efficiency in structure and function that is virtually impossible for us to duplicate. Moreover, these proteins by themselves cannot be called "living" in any sense: it is only that that they are so structured that, under the particular state of the body fluids in which they are suspended, they automatically get contorted or distorted so that they perform their particular function. Some proteins regulate movement, as in the muscle cells. Some, such as the sodium-potassium pump and hormones, regulate the body's chemical environment. Others, such as the hemoglobin molecule, have their own special functions, and so on. All these proteins regulate and interact with each other to form the special environment of a living body.

The hemoglobin protein molecule has at one end a component with just the right amount of affinity for oxygen, so that when it reaches the oxygen-rich atmosphere in the lungs, it combines with a molecule of oxygen—but when it reaches the oxygen-depleted environment of the cells, it gives the oxygen up. Simultaneously, another end of the hemoglobin molecule does the same thing for carbon dioxide, but exactly in reverse. Proteins also facilitate and control all chemical reactions in the body through enzymes. Enzymes can do this by attaching two chemicals at two ends—which then come closer to each other, thus speeding up the reaction—or by transferring energy to the reaction at one end and taking it back at the other end. Most hormones in the body—and all the super hormones, which regulate the other hormones—are proteins.

Another very important protein, which has a vital function in all cells, is the sodium-potassium, or Na^+-K^+, pump. This is a complex and very large protein found in the cell wall. It has two ends, one end projecting into and the other outside the cell. The end inside the cell has affinity for sodium and binds it, while the end outside binds potassium. The binding of the elements changes the electromechanical state of the protein, distorting its shape, which sends the sodium-containing part outside and the potassium-containing part inside. When this happens, the ends lose their stickiness and release both the sodium and potassium. This changes the molecule back to its original configuration, and it then starts another round of transporting potassium into and sodium out of the cell. So the sodium-potassium pump molecule is constantly pumping sodium outside and potassium inside the cell. Each such pumping action needs energy. This is derived from chemicals such as adenosine triphosphate (ATP), which act as the "molecular currency" of intracellular energy transfer. Such chemicals have energy-rich hydrogen bonds, which they donate wherever energy is required in chemical reactions. The spent ATP again gets recharged during the burning of glucose in the cell, when the high-energy bonds get reattached to the ATP. In this way, ATP supplies energy from glucose to all the reactions in the body.

The Na^+-K^+ pump has a very important effect because it ensures that the sodium concentration is low inside the cell compared to the outside while potassium is just the opposite, being higher inside. This difference makes the cell wall negatively charged, which keeps it in a state of electrical tension that can be set off by a number of factors, such as nerve signals. This essential property is called the *membrane potential.*

The membrane potential gives rise to all the signals in our brain and nerves, and causes our motor movements and sensory perceptions. Electrical signals in our nerves are only a movement of a wave of depolarization along the cell membrane of the nerve cells, where the cell wall during the wave becomes momentarily positive instead of negative. This positive ripple is sent from the brain to all the organs in our body through the nerves. Depolarization brought about by the ripple in the cell walls of different organs causes different effects in them. The depolarization ripple lasts only for a moment. As soon as the cell wall is depolarized, the Na^+-K^+ pump polarizes it again within microseconds.

Each brain cell consists of a cell body and an elongated process, the axon, which branches and sends signals from the cell *to* many other cells, along with several smaller processes called dendrites that bring signals *into* the cell. The dendrites of each cell receive connections from the axons of many other cells. When a cell depolarizes, its signal of depolarization flows along its axon to all the cells it connects with, and causes them to depolarize. Cells can also send signals of hyperpolarization, which makes the cell resistant to depolarization. Thus, each cell receives different signals of depolarization, neutral polarization, and hyperpolarization, at the same time. The balance of signals at any given time determines whether the cell will "fire" or not. When the signals reach a certain point, the cell will fire, sending a wave of positive polarity along its axon, which will in turn "positivize" the organs to which it connects (for example, a muscle cell). From the time it becomes active, presumably in the fetal stage, the brain is constantly buzzing with these signals running back and forth between the cells, somewhat like a controlled nuclear reaction. The system is not unlike a computer, where each brain cell is analogous to a transistor in a chip. The extremely complex connections between brain cells thus determine the processing that goes on in our minds.

Depolarization signals transmitted along the nerves cause the contraction of muscles. A nerve is nothing but a specialized axon of some cell in the brain that elongates greatly. The nerves connect the brain cells to the muscles, and when a particular brain cell depolarizes, it sends this positive wave along the nerve until it reaches its corresponding muscle fiber, where it causes depolarization of the muscle. When the muscle cell wall is depolarized, it causes a contortion in calcium receptacles inside the cells, which releases calcium ions. Inside the cells are two important protein molecules, actin and myosin. The actin rests on the myosin and is connected to it by numerous leg-like bridges. When the cell is flooded with calcium, the disturbance in the electrophysical environment causes these bridges to move, making the actin "crawl" on the myosin, much like a caterpillar. This causes muscle contraction. When the depolarization stops, the calcium withdraws and the actin reverses, causing relaxation.

Our senses also are caused by this transmission of depolarization waves, only in the opposite direction, *into* the brain. In the eye, for example, the nerve cells in the retina contain a light-sensitive chemical, rhodopsin. When rhodopsin receives light energy, it is changed into retinal acid. This change disturbs the cells' environment and causes depolarization or "positiveness" of the retinal cells, and this wave of positivity is then sent as a signal through the axons or nerves of the retinal cells back to the brain. The spent rhodopsin is re-energized in a chemical reaction regulated by other protein enzymes, which uses the energy derived from glucose brought in by blood to recharge it. Three types of retinal cells, each sensitive to a basic color—just like in a TV camera—give us color vision.

In the ear, sound energy is transmitted to special *hair cells,* which become depolarized when they are distorted mechanically. Sound waves cause this distortion when they strike the cells, and thus the signal is set up. Touch receptors in the skin send signals in the same way when pressure distorts them.

All the functions of the body can be explained in this way, simply and mechanistically. The beating of the heart, for example, is only due to some specially constituted proteins in the heart muscle cells that polarize and depolarize rhythmically as long as they are supplied with energy in the form of ATP. They will continue to beat even in a petri dish. Other functions—such as the excretory function of the kidneys, digestion, and absorption of food— are all also due to the working of different specialized proteins. The unfolding and growth of the fetus is likewise controlled entirely by the production of different proteins in a predetermined sequence by the DNA in our chromosomes.

In this way, modern science has shown that all the functions of the body are actually systematic and straightforward, and are carried out by simple chemical structures, such as proteins. At present, all functions of the body—except, perhaps, the working of the mind—have been shown to be purely mechanical. There is no need of a supernatural solution, such as the soul, to explain them. In the case of the brain, the basics of the pathways and the manner of functioning—that is, the "hardware"—is already known; it is only the "software" that remains to be deciphered. We can rest assured that scientists will one day be able to unravel much of the way our brains think. Here, too, there is no place for the soul to step in; there certainly seems to be no juncture where the brain could interact with such a "ghost" in order to produce thoughts. If the body itself can explain all aspects of physical life satisfactorily, then the theory of the soul can no longer be sustained. The soul as an explanation is unnecessary now, in the light of our present knowledge.

But if there is no soul, then all religious duties and exhortations become meaningless. If we are the body alone, there is no immortality for us, as there is nothing that will continue to exist after the body dies. Trying for rewards to obtain an eternal life then becomes absurd. All religious doctrines fall apart when confronted with this modern view of our existence, as the presence of the soul was vital for their purpose. The collapse of the concept of the soul presents a virtually insurmountable barrier for these age-old beliefs.

The knowledge of the world that we have at the beginning of the twenty-first century is vastly different from what we thought at the beginning of the nineteenth century and preceding ages. These two hundred years have completely changed our understanding of the world. In the past, the world seemed a vast, mysterious place with much that was unknown and much that was grand and harmonic, and it was natural to interpolate a powerful deity who endowed the universe with all its magical properties. Hence, practically all of metaphysics and philosophy up to that time is directed toward such a theory.

However, our present knowledge makes this position much less tenable. Although much remains to be learned, by and large the knowledge we have of the world shows it to be a vast and complex place ruled by thousands of factors, and our own lives and consciousness seem to be merely sparks from within this chaos.

In light of this knowledge, there is little place for the God of traditional metaphysics. There is now no role for a God in creation, or sustenance of life, or as a governing factor in the tumult of the cosmos. Traditional religious doctrines are unable to keep up with developments in scientific knowledge unless they abandon their fundamental roots. Almost all religions that have survived do so by turning a deaf ear to science and pretending not to have heard any of it, or by refusing to get into any arguments with scientists, maintaining that humans in some way need religion and therefore it does not matter if their teachings are incompatible with science. It has now become a widely accepted idea that religion is contradictory to science and that to follow a religion one must give it the indulgence of not opposing it with scientific facts. This is an unacceptable position to any intelligent thinker, and such views have led to the weakening of religion as a whole.

Even as these new scientific discoveries were challenging all established religions, one religious philosophy not only accepted these theories but was actually supported by them. As Darwin's theory of evolution posed its challenge to prevailing worldviews, practically all philosophies had to change drastically. In India, however, Swami Vivekananda (1863–1902), the influential proponent of the philosophies of Advaita Vedanta and Yoga, not only welcomed the theory of evolution but began to teach it himself, as he saw how it fit in with Hindu philosophy. Although Darwin's theory was far different from the Hindu idea, evolution had always been a part of Hinduism, and hence there was no contradiction. Similarly, physiological discoveries about the human body also seemed to actually follow the views propounded in the Upanishads, core scriptures of Vedantic Hinduism. The mechanical explanation of the human body and the lack of any definable soul were not contradictory to the Advaitic idea. Concepts such as the organization of the body, the transmission of energy through the nerves, and the centers for the senses and the mind, accord well with Hindu concepts about the physical body.

But it is in the relativity theory and quantum physics that Advaitism finds its clearest vindication. The idea of observer-related falsity of the world in Advaita was not properly understood even in India, and was considered by many to be only a play on words. But after Einstein, some of the Upanishadic *slokas,* or verses, seem almost like definitions of relativity. Similarly, the contradictory qualities at the heart of our existence, proposed by quantum mechanics, conform well to the Advaita philosophy. Other more recent discoveries in science seem to be leading us even further into understanding our existence in the direction described by the world's most ancient philosophers.

This complete change in our outlook in the last two hundred years means that we are now forced to re-examine our philosophies—and when we do so, most are found irreconcilable with our present knowledge. As we step into a new era, the Advaitic system remains the only spiritual philosophy that is not only not negated but actually vindicated by modern science.

4

The Origins of Indian Thought

As the sun rises up, it verily sings the Udgitha song for all creatures.
As it rises up, it dispels darkness and fear.
He who has this knowledge, surely dispels darkness and fear.

—Chandogya Upanishad I.iii.1

Any attempt to understand ourselves must begin with the question as to how it all began, and its concomitant inquiry, how it will all end. There are no final answers as yet to these questions, but our knowledge has progressed to a point where we can understand to a large extent how the universe began, how the earth began, and so on—up to the point where we finally begin our individual journeys.

The different sciences have arrived at tentative answers to these issues. None of the details are settled beyond question, but there seems little reason to doubt the whole progress of our knowledge. The scientific method of gathering data and then finding a logical interconnection between them is a vastly superior method of advancing knowledge than sitting in an armchair and thinking out solutions, which seems to be the method of most religious doctrines. Unless such religions can come out with some data to support their theories of things like creation and souls, there is no reason why we should believe them in preference over something logical and rational.

Understanding how the universe began is the realm of the science of cosmology. The most accepted answer to this at present is that it began with the big bang. The big bang is the theory that the entire universe was compressed to a single core at one time, which suddenly exploded about twelve billion years ago. This theory was arrived at after astronomers found that all the galaxies in the universe were moving away from each other. The galaxies themselves do not expand internally, because they are held together by gravitation.

When this expansion of the universe is traced backwards in time, we arrive at the conclusion that at one point, the entire universe must have been contracted to a point. This point is named a "singularity." Physicists do not know anything of what happened at the time of the explosion, but they have been able to form a number of theories regarding the manner in which the universe would have expanded—for example, what would have been the nature of the initial gases and so on.

It is important to understand that the big bang does not mean matter expanding to fill an empty universe; rather, it is the expansion of the universe itself, along with space and time, which are the real agents of the expansion. Before that, there was no universe, only the singularity. Hence, there is no central point in the universe as the site of the explosion. All the points in the universe are moving away from each other, as if new space is being generated everywhere. This is compared to the surface of a balloon being blown up, in which two points drawn anywhere on it will always be separating, without any points approaching each other. It is impossible to conceive in our minds what all this actually means and we cannot form any corresponding analogy. It must remain a theoretical conception beyond our imagination.

The big bang is very interesting to physicists, because it gives them a lot of work to do in terms of understanding the states of matter at the beginning, their temperatures, and so on. But it does not solve any of the basic questions that occur in an open inquiry. What does it really mean when we say that the universe was condensed to a point? What does "existence" signify, if the universe could also exist in such a manner that we and all the world could exist in a state of such infinite compression? What does the singularity mean, what is the nature of the "existence" of this singularity? What caused this singularity to expand, and what happened prior to this explosion?

These questions must be answered as science tries to answer the question of the first moment, and here physics changes into metaphysics, as scientists try to grapple with the basic meaning of entities like the universe, matter, and the time-space continuum. If science can answer this question, it will have answered all the questions of metaphysics too, and conversely, the answers given in the metaphysical philosophies of different religions would become as important to scientists.

Once we leave behind questions of this initial state, the sequence is not so difficult to imagine. We can conceive of the universe cooling down from its first intensely hot state and coalescing into galaxies, stars, and solar systems. The earth condensed into existence about five billion years back, and life is believed to have begun one billion years later.

It is almost impossible to conceptualize the mind-boggling lengths of time involved. Our minds often trick us into not truly understanding what such immense periods of time can mean, and the further back a stretch is, the shorter in proportion we imagine it to be. Of the four billion (or four thousand million) years of life, the first three billion (or three-fourths) of the time was represented only by single-celled organisms, beginning from the most primitive self-replicating chemicals to higher forms capable of producing their own food.

Multi-celled invertebrates appeared about one billion (or one thousand million) years ago in the sea. Life on land occupies only a half-billion, or five hundred million years. Of this five hundred million, the first humanoids occupy only the last five million years. Of this, modern anatomical humans appeared only a hundred thousand years back. Known human history, in terms of named persons and events, is only five thousand years old.

> *He hath laid down his vital germ within these worlds. He*
> *stirs with life in wombs dissimilar in kind, born as a Lion*
> *or a loudly-bellowing Bull: Vaisvanara immortal with*
> *wide-reaching might, bestowing goods and wealth on him*
> *who offers gifts.*
>
> —Rig Veda, 3.2

The first life is believed to have appeared quite early, when the earth was still in a very hot and unstable state, at a time when the atmosphere was contracting. This provided an ideal state—with tremendous activity going on and everything being subjected to intense energy bombardment—for the production of the first organic chemicals, and eventually the first self-replicating chemicals, the first life.

The first life originated in the sea, and remained there for a very long time. There is of course no record of these first puzzling chemicals at the beginning of life, but there are fossils of traces of the first recognizable life forms about three billion years back from areas once under the sea. Chemical studies of soils and rocks also detect chemicals that could only have been produced by biological processes. Soon the sea had a rich life density, although it was all of primitive, unicellular organisms.

This biological activity, coupled with the natural changes of the earth, eventually made the atmosphere an oxidizing one, and life made this huge shift from surviving in a reducing atmosphere to an oxidizing one about two billion years back. The first fossils of invertebrates in the sea are found only about eight hundred to a thousand million years back, and soon the sea had a very great diversity of life forms. Once life made this change from single-celled to multi-celled organisms there was a rapid diversification and colonization of new areas, because of the advantages of such forms. Sexual reproduction was another watershed that allowed for a much more rapid rate of evolution. The first life on land appeared about 450 million years back.

On land, species multiplied rapidly and in amazing varieties. The dinosaurs came and went about sixty-five million years back, and from then on it was the era of mammals, until, about five million years ago, we find the first hominids.

Humans and other primates such as gorillas and chimpanzees had a common line of descent until about five to ten million years back, when they began to diverge from a common ancestor. This common ancestor had several lines of descent, leading to other primates like the apes but with one special line leading to the hominids. Hence it is not that man evolved from monkeys but that monkeys, gorillas, chimpanzees, and man all had one common ancestor far back in time. From this common link evolved humanoids, "gorrilloids," "chimpanzoids," and so on. Ever since, these species have all been diverging from each other.

Of the different humanoids, only the most efficient type, *Homo sapiens*, survived, and it pushed the other descendants into extinction by virtue of its overwhelming superiority. Similarly, of the "gorilloids" only the most efficient two or three species of gorillas survived, and so on. The common ancestor was not a half gorilla-half human but something probably quite different and much smaller, like a tree shrew. It has not been possible to trace this ancestor—the missing link—and the immediate lines of descent from it because of a paucity of fossils in the period from five to ten million years ago. Of all the descendants of this ancestor, we find today only a few of the primate species, including humans, who are best-adapted to the present environment. Still, members of some of the ape species such as gorillas appear headed toward extinction even without the intervention of humans.

From around five million years back, we find the fossils of the first humans, the hominids called *Australopithecus*. They were as yet very similar to apes in almost all respects, but had two very important distinguishing features: bipedalism, or the ability to walk upright, and an increased cranial cavity, which meant a larger brain. Bipedalism was important because it freed the hands, which could then be used very efficiently for a variety of functions such as hunting, tool-making, food gathering, and other fine work. Once the hand did not have the primary function of locomotion, it also adapted by forming the opposable thumb, which in humans can be pressed against all the other fingers, and which is vital for fine work. Intelligence was important for better hunting techniques, better tool-making, better shelter construction, and information sharing.

The hominids continued to evolve, and about 2.5 million years ago they formed the species *Homo habilis*, which evolved further around 1.5 million years ago to give rise to *Homo erectus*. These were progressively more human-like, if still rather nasty looking. All these first evolutionary steps took place in Africa, until *Homo erectus* started the first human migration and spread all over Asia and Europe, so that humans now occupied the major part of the globe around one million years back.

About two hundred thousand years ago the next major step took place, with the evolution of *Homo sapiens* from *Homo erectus*. The *Homo sapiens* species comprised a number of subspecies—such as *H. sapiens neanderthalis*, the Neanderthal man, and *H. sapiens sapiens*, the modern man—in different parts of the world. These different subspecies evolved from different groups of *H. erectus* in different geographical regions and spread out, so that by a hundred thousand years ago we find a number of *H. sapiens* subspecies ruling over the world. But by thirty thousand years back we find only one subspecies in control, the *Homo sapiens sapiens*, or modern humans, all other subspecies having died out.

How this subspecies, *Homo sapiens sapiens*, evolved and came to dominate so completely over the other species of *Homo sapiens* (such as *Homo sapiens neanderthalis*) that they became extinct is a subject of controversy. There are two competing theories among anthropologists about this. In the "Out of Africa" model, it is believed that *H. sapiens sapiens* evolved in only one place somewhere in Africa and from there migrated out to the world, making this the second migration after the *Homo erectus* one million years previously. They were so superior to the other subspecies such as *Homo sapiens neanderthalis* that, along with changes in the environment, they drove them to extinction, not through actual fighting but through competition for scarce resources. The other subspecies, such as the Neanderthal man, had no role in the evolution of modern humans.

In the "Multi-Regional" model, it is believed that *H. sapiens sapiens* evolved as a whole from all the other different subspecies such as the Neanderthal man in different areas of the world with a great deal of interbreeding, and all the subspecies became subsumed in this new form. Recent findings, both genetic and archaeological, seem to support the "Out of Africa" model.

Why did only one species develop intelligence, and why did the other primates (and in fact all other species) remain so atrophied in their intelligence? The answer is probably that intelligence does not automatically guarantee better survival. Many experiments as well as anecdotal stories prove that gorillas and chimpanzees have quite a high degree of intelligence, equal to that of a four-year-old child. But this has not helped them in dominating their environment in the wild in terms of ensuring a better food supply, better shelter, or protection. Their survival capabilities are not much better than other animals in their environment. Intelligence is not a homogenous factor but comprises a number of skills such as memory, increased motor skills, communication, and imagination. All the different skills are interconnected and need to be equally developed before they begin to have an effect.

Hence, there is probably a threshold level that intelligence has to cross before it actually helps in survival, and once this threshold is crossed, intelligence becomes a real factor and begins to develop rapidly. In humans, perhaps this threshold was crossed in a particular field by, say, improved communication skills through better vocalization, and it would have been only when this particular skill had developed that development in other fields such as increased memory would begin to help. Thus, once the threshold was crossed with any one skill, it would start off a cascade of development of intelligence as a whole. In other animals, this chance event of an isolated skill crossing the threshold never happened, and so the whole cascade never took off.

Human intelligence has been without doubt the main factor behind our dominance, besides other things like free hands. Fire was being used as early as one million years ago by *H. erectus*, and tools were being made with ever-increasing sophistication right from the first hominids. Around fifty thousand years ago, there was a big increase in human population and dominance over the environment, and it is widely theorized that this was due to the development of a sophisticated language, which would have given an immense boost to progress.

An important feature in the evolution of humans has been the role of the ice ages. The ice ages are periods in earth's history when much of the land is covered by huge sheets of ice. In fact in scientific terms we are still in an ice age that began about two million years ago, and this is just a warm interval beginning from around ten thousand years back. During cold periods of the ice age, as water becomes trapped in ice, the water levels recede and land bridges open up, which allows for migration and interbreeding. During warm periods, the bridges are again flooded, isolating human groups and at the same time providing a suitable climate for increases in population.

The two main migrations from Africa, the first of *Homo erectus* and the second of *Homo sapiens sapiens*, are also believed to have occurred during ice ages. This immensely complex interplay between humans and the earth; the changes in human development that were by turns aided and impeded by climate changes;

and the periods of isolation, growth, and migration of different groups of humans at different times are all like so many chapters in the long story of human evolution, which are as yet far from being fully understood.

> *Then he drinks it saying, "The radiant sun is adorable—the winds are blowing sweetly, the rivers are shedding honey, may the herbs be sweet unto us!*
> *Swaha to the earth.*
> *Glory we meditate upon; May the nights and days be charming, and the dust of the earth be sweet, may heaven, our father, be gracious!*
> *Swaha to the sky."*

—Brihadaranyaka Upanishad, VI.iii.6

The real development of human civilization as we know it now began about ten thousand years back at the beginning of the present warm interval. As the ice receded, vast parts of the world came out of the cold and enjoyed a climate suitable and comfortable for us. There was a proliferation of human population, and newer settlements came into being. With the development of agriculture, there was the beginning of settled life and big advancements in culture. Civilization as we know it today can be said to have begun about five thousand years ago, around three thousand BCE, with the Bronze Age civilizations.

The Bronze Age is so called because bronze was one of the main materials used for tools, weapons, and other objects. Bronze is mainly copper mixed with some tin, and it came to be the first metal to be used because it melted easily, and hence could be extracted with much cruder techniques. When techniques for extracting iron came to be known, it came to be used preferentially because it was far more readily available and much harder, giving rise to the Iron Age.

The Bronze Age represented a coming of age for humanity, and it marked the end of years of semi-wild existence and the beginning of the sophisticated culture, language, and wisdom of human civilization. The Bronze Age is one of the most intriguing passages of human history. The civilizations of this age still retained contact with the most ancient traditions of nature worship, and subscribed to many mysterious rites and rituals. At the same time, they appear to have been very advanced in some areas of their knowledge and left us beguiling archaeological wonders and literary achievements whose full significance is not yet known.

Another surprising aspect is the apparent interconnections of these civilizations. The Bronze Ages left us Stonehenge in Britain, the pyramids in Egypt, the Vedas and the Indo-Saraswati cities in India, the temples in Mesopotamia, and legends of Minotaurs and magic in Aegean Greece. Other strange remains are the huge stone faces of the Cook Islands and the much later Mayan civilization. The baffling nature of these remains, the almost superhuman technology that many of them must have needed and that seems to have been lost in the subsequent Iron Ages, and, most importantly, the apparent close links that existed between different civilizations at that time that are only being discovered now, present a beguiling mystery and have given rise to a number of legends, including that of Atlantis, to explain it.

The Atlantis theory proposes that a much superior civilization had existed about ten thousand years back, and it was the Atlanteans who taught the people of the Bronze Age their science. Another theory is that aliens from outer space came to Earth at that time and gave this technology. Whatever the actual truth may be, the bizarre nature of such theories do point to the great mystery of the Bronze Age and show that much remains to be known about this period before we can claim to have a thorough knowledge of human progress.

It was probably during this period that the source of all Hindu thought, the Vedas, were composed, but this is still controversial. All Hindus today trace their roots to these Vedas, but in modern historical interpretation, there are two opposing views regarding the people, the time of their composition, and the geographical site. This controversy, ironically, has nothing to do with India itself; it arose from a vicious theory that had its origin in Europe and that gave rise to the calamitous events of World War II. This is the theory of Aryanism that proposes that a race called Aryans spread and conquered the whole world around 1500 BCE, and that all modern culture originated from them. It arose from a twisted reconstruction of Indian and European history by Europeans when they first came across the Vedas.

It is surprising now to think that before the eighteenth century the word "Aryan" was unknown in Europe. The only people who called themselves Aryan were Indians. The Persians of old in Iran had also called themselves Aryan, but after their conversion to Islam this became a forgotten part of their history. When the Vedas and other Sanskrit texts were first translated into European languages around the 1750s, many were amazed by the richness revealed in them. It was soon realized that there was great deal in common between Sanskrit and Latin, and the theory arose that the two languages had developed from a common source.

For a time, this source was believed to be India itself, and thinkers of that time such as Voltaire began to consider India as their ancient motherland and the source of all the wisdom of European civilization. But around the beginning of the nineteenth century, this interpretation began to change. This was brought about mainly due to a rise of ultra-nationalism among German philosophers. The common language theory was carried forward to mean a common race too, but it was twisted around so that the Germans became the true Aryans; Indians, ironically, became a side branch of this master race, although until a few years previously Germans had hardly known the word "Aryan," which was an ancient birthright to Indians. A German scholar, Max Mueller, had concluded from a rather nonsensical study of the differences in the parts of the Vedas that Sanskrit had originated around 1500 BCE. This became a part of the lore of the master race to give rise to the Aryan theory in its full glory—the master race that conquered the world in 1500 BCE, and gave rise to a new world.

The distinguishing features of this race were of course their anatomical features, which came to represent the type of tall, blonde, white people. The Aryans were also supposedly characterized by the use of horses, and along with their use of iron in arrows and spears, the final image was of these warlike people conquering the Bronze Age world on their horses and chariots with iron weapons, thus bringing in the tougher, more "masculine" Iron Age in their wake. These people supposedly set up the Indian, Greek, and Persian civilizations and hence were the originators of the world civilization of today.

This distorted theory was now used to interpret Indian history, and the Vedas became the literature of this master race that entered India in 1500 BCE. When the archaeological remains of an ancient Bronze Age civilization in India from around 3500 BCE to 2000

BCE were discovered, the Indo-Saraswati civilization, this was fitted into the theory to show that this civilization had been an old degenerate Bronze Age civilization that was conquered by the victorious Aryans. Only the later Gangetic civilization, around 1000 BCE, was considered to be a true Aryan civilization.

This interpretation of the Vedic people was quite alien to the Indians. The Indians had always called themselves Aryans, and their understanding of the Vedas—their ancient myths, songs, and culture—had always told them that it was in this land that they had been settled since time immemorial, and that it was here that the Vedas were composed.

The Indo-Saraswati civilization, which is pre-1500 BCE, shows a civilization of numerous cities with kings and priests, and it conforms to the legends of sages, kings, and priests of Vedic lore. Due to some environmental factors, mainly the drying up of the Saraswati River, the Indo-Saraswati civilization had to be abandoned to give rise to the Gangetic civilization, which conforms to the Puranic and epic times, when the Puranas and the epics were written. This is how most Indians still understand their history, even when they have been taught otherwise in schools and colleges.

The Aryan theory, on the other hand, made the Vedic people (the people described in the Vedas) into a nomadic, semi-barbaric people, the true Aryans, who composed the Vedas in an alien land and whose contact with India began only much later. According to Mueller, the Vedic culture therefore is not one grown organically in the present homeland of the Hindus, and Indians of today are only a mixture of Aryans, or the "pure" Vedic people, and the tribes they defeated.

The Gods possessed the wealth bestowing Agni. Praise him, ye
Aryan folk, as chief performer of sacrifice, Adored and ever
toiling, Well-tended, Son of Strength, the Constant Giver.

—Rig Veda, 1.96.

The theory of "Aryan invasion" and migration is so riddled with
aberrations that no historian today outside of India will extend
full-hearted support to it. It is ironic that while everywhere else
the Aryan theory is considered a part of fascist propaganda, in
India itself it is just the reverse. Left-wing opinion-makers support it and call those who oppose it fascists! In the first place, there
is no archaeological evidence whatsoever of such a movement of
people into India at that time. When there is any significant movement of people, they always leave behind signs such as new styles
of pottery, tools, and ornaments, but no such remains have been
found in India.

The Aryan theory mainly counted on an interpretation of the
writings of the Vedas for proof, but this interpretation has now
been roundly challenged. The various passages that were once
quoted in support of an invasion have been logically shown to
have other interpretations as well. For example, the descriptions of
pastoral life in the earliest Vedas could just as well be those of the
pre-urban phase of the cities, and the fights between *Dasas* (non-
Aryan tribes) and Aryans could be fights between the city dwellers
of the Indo-Saraswati period and the surrounding tribesmen, or
even allude to battles between different cities.

Another important point is that archeological evidence of bull-
worship, fire altars, and other rituals mentioned in the Vedas have
been found in the cities of the Indo-Saraswati period. An impartial

view should have no difficulty in identifying the descriptions of the Indo-Saraswati cities in the Vedic hymns.

The clinching piece of evidence is the discovery, fairly recently, of a dry bed of a very large river, parts of which are still known as the Saraswati, and the discovery of numerous cities of that period on its banks. The Vedas do not mention the Ganges (or Ganga River, as it is known in India), and its chief rivers are the Indus and the Saraswati. Clearly, this fits in very nicely with the Indo-Saraswati civilization being the Vedic civilization. This river has been shown geologically to have dried up around 2000 BCE, and it was this perhaps that compelled the people to move into the Ganga valley. The Aryans, who were supposed to have come in at 1500 BCE, would have found only a dry bed. It takes a very dogmatic mind to believe that they would compose the hymns of the Vedas in praise of a dry river!

There are many other points that go against the Aryan theory. In the first place, the mythical homeland of the Aryans has not been found yet. It is proposed to have been in all kinds of places ranging from central Asia to the Caspian Sea, but there is no evidence, archaeological or otherwise, of such a civilization. In fact, one theory even proposes that the earth is hollow and the Aryans came from a superior civilization that still exists underneath our feet! There are also the usual suspects like Atlantis and space aliens.

These out-of-the-way theories are just about as credible as any of the others proposed. Again, nomadic civilizations by their very nature are thinly populated and spread out, and this means that, without exception, they have been found to have somewhat primitive cultures. It is very unlikely therefore that a nomadic group would develop sophisticated and multi-textured languages like Sanskrit and Latin. The theory of the Aryans being an Iron Age people who brought iron into India would in fact contradict their being the Vedic people, because most of the Vedas are quite clearly Bronze Age texts. It is also ridiculous to propose that anyone would drive in chariots over the mountain passes of Afghanistan.

This leads us to the problem of horses, the one point most often quoted by Aryan theorists. Horses are very frequently mentioned in the Vedas, but little archaeological evidence of horses has been uncovered in the Indo-Saraswati cities. This has been cited to show that these cities cannot be those of the Vedas. It is not that no equine bones have been found—in fact they have been found in large numbers—but they were all described by the early colonial archaeologists as "unstratified," "badly recorded," or "onager bones," the thrice-condemned! The now-rare, mysterious onager, or wild ass, was apparently quite common then and used to wander about the cities like a stray animal.

Some unequivocal evidence of horses *has* been found in the cities, although it is relatively scarce. The important point is that the horse problem cuts both ways, because horse bones begin to be found in significant numbers in India only around the fourth century BCE, thus ruling out the presence of any horse-riding people before that.

The Aryan theory also had its problems in its interpretations of other histories. In Europe, the first major civilization, the Aegean civilization of the Greek island of Crete was considered a non-Aryan, non-Greek-speaking, and Bronze Age civilization that was conquered by the Aryan race in 1500 BCE. The difficulties associated with this have been a subject of controversy since then.

There is again no archaeological evidence to show that the later Greeks were an entirely different people from the Aegeans. Besides, the script of the Myceneans of ancient Greece, Linear B, is only a derivation of that of the Aegeans, and because the Greek script has been deciphered, there is no reason to doubt that the Aegean script will also be a Greek one when it is figured out.

Another problem is that posed by the Persians, who appeared in Iran at the end of the Mesopotamian civilization. The Persians used Sanskrit as their official language and also called themselves Aryans, and it is very likely that they were the westernmost part of the Indo-Saraswati civilization, as there is clear archaeological evidence of the civilization extending through Afghanistan into Iran.

The Persians may have moved out after wars with the mainland Indo-Saraswati cites. It is significant that they called their gods *ahura* or *asura* (asura has come to mean "demon" in Sanskrit), and their god is Ahura Mazda, "the great asura." Their evil ones are called *devas* (deva means "god" in Sanskrit)—just the opposite of the Vedas.

A better theory, which is consistent with the latest findings in archaeology as well as genetic information and literary interpretation, is that South Asians and Europeans had indeed originated from the same source and then separated, but this separation was much earlier than 1500 BCE, much earlier than the Bronze Age even, at a time after the ices had melted when there was a common ancestral group that were the progenitors of all Aryans. This group then migrated and separated into two or more groups, and their respective peoples shaped the Bronze Age civilizations: the Indo-Saraswati (Vedic) civilization, in India, and the Aegean civilization, in Greece. These same civilizations developed in the Iron Age into the Gangetic and Greek civilizations, respectively.

Such a theory would agree not only with scientific evidence, but also with the myths and traditions of ancient Indians and Greeks. The Aryan theory has already been used to justify one of the saddest episodes of human history. It is vital now that this theory should be subjected to very close examination, and its truth or falsity be cleared up once and for all, so that we can once again look at our history with open minds.

The Indo-Saraswati civilization comprised a large number of cities on the banks of the Indus and Saraswati rivers in the northwestern part of what is now modern-day India. It was a Bronze Age civilization, its full development ranging from around 3500 BCE to 2000 BCE. It was concurrent with the Egyptian, Mesopotamian, and Aegean civilizations. At that time, it was the largest of all its contemporary civilizations in both geography and population.

The civilization is curious in character. There is none of the flamboyance that marked its contemporaries in its sculpture and design. Instead we have some very well-planned cities with row upon row of similar brick houses set along straight streets with excellent sewage facilities and covered drains, huge granaries, common religious places with the fire altars mentioned in the Vedas, and a very successful trading system. It offered the greatest civic amenities to its citizens and was without doubt the most democratic of the civilizations of that time, which were generally characterized by palaces amid surrounding hovels. It was as if a very intelligent people had sat down and planned out how to build great cities that would benefit everyone, not just the rich or the rulers.

Religion undoubtedly formed a very big role in this ordered society, and a large portion of space was set aside for it. In the seals of the cities we find motifs that are still a part of Hinduism today: the great Bull, the peepul tree, a man in a Yogic posture, the swastika, and images of the Mother Goddess, Shiva, and other deities. The ideas and words of this ancient civilization continue to reverberate throughout Indian society today with the strength of their simplicity and applicability to modernity.

The Indian civilization, along with the Chinese, still retains its direct links with the Bronze Age. Hindus still follow basically the same religious rites that we see depicted in the ancient seals; the cow-worship and other myths and traditions of the Vedas are still living forms. In most other civilizations, there has been a sharp break between the ancient and the modern. The Indian and Chinese provide examples of two civilizations where the spiritual culture has developed continuously through the ages, and it is no surprise that today they have the largest populations in the world. They are separated by the highest mountains in the world, the Himalayas. It is remarkable how effective this separation has been, with hardly any major cultural links between these two neighbors, the only exception being the migration of Buddhism from India to China.

The image that India conjures up in many people today is that of a vast and illiterate people living in poverty and practicing a somewhat strange and superstitious religion. But this was not always the case. It might be surprising to realize that until the 1700s, India was in fact known for its wisdom and wealth, before two hundred years of colonial rule destroyed much of it. The wealth of India was legendary, and drew merchants and adventurers from all over the world. It was this wealth that drew Columbus to find a sea route to India, although in a huge miscalculation he landed in the "West Indies." It was also this wealth that made India the most sought-after goal for colonial rule, and many desperate battles followed for it. When it was finally conquered by the British, the Indian subcontinent was one of the, if not *the*, richest region in the world. Two hundred years later, when it became free, it was one of the poorest countries in the world.

*Even while lying in the womb, I came to know the birth of all
the gods.*

*A hundred iron citadels held me down. Then, like a hawk, I
forced my way through by dint of the knowledge of the Self.*

—Aitareya Upanishad II.i.5

India has always been famous for its wisdom, through the strength
of its philosophical systems and theoretical science in such branches
as mathematics. Travelers have come in all ages in search of this
"wisdom of the East," from Pythagoras and many other Europeans to the Chinese and other Asian people. This wealth is contained in the vast ancient literature of India.

The root of all this knowledge is the Vedas. From this knowledge sprang the Puranas, the Agama texts, and the epics. Based
loosely on these is a fantastic array of texts, covering every aspect
of philosophical intercourse possible in its minutest details. There
are also huge collections of texts covering subjects ranging from
very advanced books on the sciences, such as mathematics, economics, administration, and medical and veterinary practices, to
treatises on arts such as music and dance, as well as bewitching
literary pieces such as plays and poetry. There are also intriguing
texts like the Kama Sutra, a text on sexuality, and any number of
books on magic. Much of this knowledge continues to be as relevant today as when it was first thought out.

The Vedas form the fountainhead of this wisdom. Most of the
subsequent texts draw upon it for authority, even when they deal
with entirely new subjects. The Vedas are not one book but a huge
collection of books, almost like a library in itself. This library may
be said to have four walls, containing the four Vedas: the Rig,

Shyam, Jajur, and the Atharva. Each wall may be said to have four shelves containing the four parts of each Veda: the Samhita, the Brahmana, the Aranyaka, and the Upanishads, with each shelf containing a large number of books.

The Samhita of each Veda is the collection of hymns, and each Samhita has several books; the Rig Samhita, for example, contains ten books. Below this are the Brahmanas, which each contain several books that contain descriptions of ritualistic worship, the Vedic *yagna*, or fire ceremonies.

Next come the Aranyakas, which describe in detail the exact mode of performance of the yagnas, the size of the altars, the chants to be said, and so on. These yagnas are often extremely complex, requiring huge quantities of things like milk, sandalwood, the donation of cows and other gifts, and the participation of a large number of priests, each with their specified function. These yagnas continue until the present day in a very simplified form, and the burning of a fire altar is still a must for important Hindu occasions like births, marriages, and deaths.

In the last shelf we have the books of the Upanishads, which contain the philosophical knowledge of the Vedas. The Upanishads form the core wisdom of the Vedas. The other books are mainly to do with primitive nature worship, and philosophies based on them could not survive for long. Vedic philosophy today usually refers to Upanishadic philosophy alone.

The Upanishads are also called the Vedantas (from *anta*, meaning "end"), because they come at the end of the Vedas. The knowledge contained in them was considered to be so esoteric that it was also called the *forest philosophy* or the *secret philosophy*, because only sages and *rishis* were capable of understanding it. The books contain only several short aphorisms, called *sutras*, which are by themselves so enigmatic that they can be made to support many different philosophies.

The Upanishads are explained by different scholars in their commentaries on the sutras, and depending on the persuasion of the scholars, the sutras are made to support different streams of philosophy. Hence the Upanishads have been interpreted to derive the three main forms of Vedantic Hinduism today: the dualistic, the qualified monistic, and the monistic or Advaitic.

The main wisdom of the Upanishads have been collected into a single book, the Brahma Sutras, but this book is as enigmatic as the remainder of the text, if not more so, and its sutras too are as fiercely fought over, with commentators of the three schools giving different interpretations of each of the sutras right from the first sutra itself: "Now, therefore, this inquiry of Brahman [is taken up]." This innocuous-looking beginning is enough to start off a huge debate, and from the commentary on this sutra alone the different positions are taken up. The final form of the three Upanishadic philosophies as we know them now were given only in the period from the eighth to tenth centuries, by Shankara-charya, Ramanuja, and Madhava.

In the Vedas, the main rivers are the Indus and the Saraswati. But as this basin dried up, the Gangetic valley became the center of Indian civilization, and led to the renewal of Indian religious thought. The scriptures composed here depend on the Vedas in terms of their overall development. This was contemporary with the Greek civilization, which had by this time supplanted the Aegean.

The religious books that are the most widely known in India today are undoubtedly the two epics, the *Ramayana* and the *Mahabharata*. The two stories are in verse form and are the longest epics in world literature, surpassing by far the Iliad and Odyssey, with which they bear many resemblances. They are set on the banks of the Ganga (or Ganges) River and tell of an idyllic period of Indian life, with their portrayal of the epitome of heroism, self-sacrifice, and philosophical wisdom in the lives of the main characters. These two epics have influenced virtually every aspect of Indian culture, and stories and philosophy from them rule over the daily practice of religion.

These epics have given us the two warrior gods of India—Rama, or Ram, and Krishna—and their stories have since become the main features of Hindu religious life. The *Ramayana* is the story of Ram, and uses the study of his life as he battles with evil to act as a guide in all matters of daily life. The *Mahabharata* is a complex story of two families of cousins who fight a war against each other, and has a vast repository of short tales and philosophical wisdom interspersed into the main text. Krishna was the main general of this war, where he sided with the good forces of the Pandavas.

This epic also contains the Bhagavad Gita, the root text of Hinduism, which contains teachings used to delineate all the major philosophies of India. By now we already find the concept of India, or Bharat, as a single country. The text describes how all the kings of the different parts of the country—from Assam (or Kamrup, as it was known at that time) in the north to the Pandyas, Kerelas, and Chola kings in the south—gather together in the two opposing camps on the battlefield for the biggest feud of the times.

Besides the epics, the other important religious texts of this period are the Agama texts, which support the Tantric and Shaivite philosophies. These texts do not quote the Vedas for authority, but in terms of their overall domain they are very much a derivation of the Vedas. The Puranas, with their fantastic tales of gods and goddesses and their doings, set the tone for future religious worship. The Vaishnavite texts, which extol the worship of Lord Vishnu mainly in his form as the avatar Krishna, also came to be composed around this time. All this religious literature was concomitant with developments in many other spheres of science and arts, and a large number of texts on these subjects continued to be written right down to modern times.

Practically all these texts were composed in Sanskrit, but from around the first century CE another important source of Indian civilization began to develop in the south. The texts of this civilization, the *sangam* literature, were in Tamil. They were composed in three sangams, (or conclaves) of people with gods who, by tradition, came in from the seas about ten thousand years ago (quite interestingly for Atlantis theorists). Furthermore, the Buddhist texts were composed in Pali rather than Sanskrit from around the third century BCE, and they are a huge collection in themselves. From around the tenth century, texts began to be composed in the other Indian languages as well, and gradually Sanskrit fell into disuse, remaining a classical language only.

All this literature adds up to a vast corpus, much of which remains untranslated and unknown today. All fields of human thought are covered in great detail, both in the sciences and the arts. The wisdom of this most ancient and large group of literature continues to reverberate in India today, and its freshness and intrinsic value continues to energize the renewal of Indian spiritual life.

5

Different Positions in Philosophy

Tell me, O Swan, your ancient tale.
From what land do you come, O Swan? To what shore do you fly?
Where will you take your rest, O Swan, and what do you seek?
This morning, O Swan, awake, arise and follow me!

—Kabir 2.24

The search for knowledge has been the most important force leading us onward in the advancement of our civilization. When we begin to look at the knowledge that is in our possession, the most important knowledge undoubtedly concerns our own selves. But it is a paradox that this is also the area where we have the greatest amount of controversy. We are unable to define our own identity, life, death, or answer the most basic questions: Where did I come from? Where will I go? Am I finite or infinite? Is it true that I came into existence only a few years ago and will cease to exist in another few years?

It seems a piquant position that we really do not know anything about our existence for sure, and it is only by *not* asking the important questions that we can get on with our lives. Our knowledge of the existence of the world is also not based on absolute foundations, and when we examine this knowledge, we keep coming up against dead ends, as in trying to determine the nature of time, space, and cause-effect relations.

The branch of philosophy that enquires into the problems regarding our existence is called metaphysics. This may be considered the core of all other systems of philosophy, because it contains the first problems that come up in philosophy. To study the different religions, we first of all need to understand their metaphysics and whether they are consistent with modern knowledge. Only when we can agree with a religion's metaphysical basis can we think of accepting its tenets. Other problems of religious philosophy such as ethics, epistemology, or the inquiry into knowledge are secondary. Hence this is the core issue that must be studied. In our struggle to understand our existence, we can define the starting point in two ways.

In *metaphysical idealism*, the starting point, prior to beginning all philosophical speculation, is taken as the existence of the knower, the "I" alone, and this existence is the base of all further enquiries. Everything else—knowledge and the objects of the world—is studied only in reference to it, and their existence is understood only in relation to the "I." In contrast to this, in *metaphysical realism*, the starting point is the *trio* of knower, knowledge, and the thing known; all three are taken to exist simultaneously and have the same level of existence and reality. The world is then analyzed from this base.

In metaphysical idealism, the initial existence of the "I," a pure form that exists prior to any experience or interaction with the world, is assumed. This is the position of most of Western philosophy. This "I"—*my mind*—then goes on to experience the world. The problem of metaphysical idealism is that, if its logic is followed strictly, it inevitably leads to solipsism. Solipsism is the proposition that nothing except the "I" exists, and everything else is unreal. Once we start with the "I" alone, then all the experiences and sensations that we are having are things that exist only in relation to "my mind;" they do not have *anything else* as their basis. We cannot know anything except through our minds. Even the things that we experience directly, the things that we see or touch, may be false. We know that in dreams we "see" things and "touch" things that we know are not really there; our minds are simply deluded into believing that they are there. Therefore it may be that even in this waking world, our minds are being deluded into thinking that these things around us exist.

The seventeeth-century French philosopher René Descartes described a demon that could cheat our minds with all these sensations of a vast world outside us. There might be such a "demon" that is feeding impressions into our mind (like the computer network in the film *The Matrix*), or it could be that the waking world is a spontaneous dream of our mind. Other people could also be simply a part of this delusion, along with everything around us. There is no way that we can show that the things that we touch, feel, or experience in any other way (i.e., the whole of the outside world), actually exist.

For example, when we see a red ball, what we actually experience is our mind sending us the information that we are seeing a red ball. We know that in a dream, we can see a red ball even when it is not actually there. So also in our "waking" state, our mind could simply be sending us this information without anything being there. Similarly, when we touch something, when we walk or talk, all that we know is that this is the information that our minds are sending to us. We do not know if there is actually an outside world with which we are interacting.

Hence when we take the initial idealistic metaphysical position of the "I" or the mind alone being the only real thing, then it is entirely possible that this whole world is untrue and nothing except I *myself*, my own mind, exists. Everything else is a big dream that *my mind* has dreamt up, or, in Descartes' view, a vision fed into my mind by a demon. The outside world cannot be shown to exist in any way from this starting point.

The other position, metaphysical realism, is the philosophy of the Upanishads. Here the knower, the knowledge, and the thing known are considered to have simultaneous existence and are equally real. The "thing known"—that is, the outside world—exists independently of the knower and the knower exists independently of the "thing known." When a particular object interacts with a particular "knower," then knowledge is produced in the knower. The attempt to understand the world is taken up from this trio as the basis, rather than from any single entity among these.

When the "I" or "my mind" alone is taken to exist first, then knowledge becomes something that exists only in reference to this "I." When everything exists only in reference to the "I," then we must ask how far the outside world, to which this knowledge purports, has influence in this knowledge. Hence epistemology (the study of how we gather knowledge) becomes very complex in the Western view. Differing views exist, from pure idealistic epistemology, which says that the outside world has no influence at all on our knowledge, to empiricist epistemology, which admits varying levels of influence of the outside world on our knowledge. However, empiricism in such a philosophy is always obstructed by the fact that we do not know in the first place if the outside world exists. Pure idealism, in which the world would be nothing more than a dream, is of course, always hard to accept.

Faced with these two positions, we may ask, why should we not begin from the standpoint of the "I" alone, metaphysical idealism, instead of the trio of knower, knowledge, and the thing that is known of metaphysical realism?

From the standpoint of Hindu philosophy, the answer is that in Hinduism, the *individual "I,"* (i.e., the "I" of the world) is inevitably associated with thoughts and sensations. It is in fact *because it is associated* with thoughts and sensations that the "I" becomes individualized from the absolute. Hence we cannot consider the individual "I" as separate from thoughts and sensations, which in turn arise from the things thought of or experienced. If the "I" existed *alone* from the very beginning, then it would not have had any thoughts or sensations, and would have been in an undifferentiated state. Therefore we cannot take the "I" as existing in a pure state without anything else; the "I" will exist only when the rest of this differentiated world exists.

Such a position is logically consistent and does not depend on doctrinal positions to make sense of the world. Metaphysical realism is our everyday, commonsense view of the world, and also underpins modern scientific views such as evolution. Modern views on consciousness also do not recognize any individual "I" apart from thoughts and sensations and assume that this "I" is a complex of thoughts and sensations.

The theory of evolution finally put paid to all concepts of metaphysical idealism. The mind did not come into existence first and then have these "ideas" about matter; rather, matter existed first and through evolution caused the formation of the mind. When we think of the mind as existing independently of matter, then everything seems puzzling and inexplicable. But this is simply because we are looking at things the wrong way. When we see them in the correct way, everything falls into place and we see that it is matter, in the shape of the environment, which has given rise to mind, and hence both are coexistent.

This is in accord with both evolutionary theory and the Indian view of the simultaneous existence of knower, knowledge, and the thing that is known. Any solipsism would have to contradict evolutionary theories, and consider them to be one more game of Descartes' demon or one more bad dream. Convoluted arguments of idealistic versus empiricist epistemology also become irrelevant in the face of evolution.

> *Willed by whom does the directed mind go towards its object?*
> *Being directed by whom does the vital force that precedes all,*
>   *proceed towards its duty? By whom is this speech willed that*
>   *people utter?*
> *Who is the effulgent being who directs the eyes and ears?*
>
> —Kena Upanishad I.i

Even after accepting that the world exists, we might ask whether this existence is in a real sense, whether the world behaves in a "natural" way, or whether it is rigidly controlled by some outside power, like Descartes' demon. When we start from idealistic metaphysics, as we have seen, this becomes an argument that is impossible to logically disprove. If the entire world is only an activity of our mind, then it is certainly possible that our minds are getting deceived by some outside intelligence, or perhaps by themselves, into having this dream of the world. All idealistic metaphysicians have to contend with this logical cul-de-sac into which their philosophy leads them.

But even from a realistic viewpoint, we may argue that although the outside world exists, it does not exist "naturally." It is rigidly controlled by some "superpower," which is putting on a show for our benefit, or to test us. This show might be something put on only for "my" individual benefit. Perhaps I am the only natural person out here and all the rest are conspiring against me. We may ask, what do we really know of the world? We know what we have experienced and what we have heard as sources of knowledge from others. But what if the whole world is a giant conspiracy and I am its victim? For example, what proof do we really have that something we hear happening in a far-off place has really happened? We have only read about it in the newspapers or seen it on the TV. What if the papers and TV were all conspirators against us trying to delude us? Similarly, all the people around us could also be conspirators who are simply playing out a script put for them!

The victims of such a conspiracy could even be the entire human race; perhaps we are all being made fools of by some giant power for its own ends. The physical things that we see or hear may also be a magic show put on for us, and maybe things look completely different when we turn our backs. This is a common proposition of some religions, which argue that a supernatural power, God, is controlling each and every event in the world, although in this case it is being done apparently with a benign view.

The vital thing about this world is that it is not running chaotically. The world and its events follow some definite laws: "For fear of Him, Fire Burns, from fear shines the sun." The ancients got their principles right; the world moves in a harmoniously interrelated fashion. The events of the world behave in an orderly fashion with definite laws *and therefore are predictable*. Hence it would be impossible for any supernatural force to be controlling the world at its whim, as it would be entirely governed by laws that it would have to follow. In the toss of a coin, for example, there is a fifty-fifty chance of either face showing up. Because there are such a large number of factors pulling in different directions, the contrary pulls eventually cancel out and so in a large number of turns, the results are approximately even. It is because there is no controlling factor for the fall of the coin that there is an equal chance of either of the two faces showing.

It may be argued that it is perhaps still an outside force that is controlling the coin, only in its devious way it ensures that the probability laws are being followed. The end result is the same: as long as the force has to follow the laws it means that it does not have control over the coin, and it also is controlled by the laws. In an infinite number of such events as the movement of planets or formation of galaxies, or even in such things as which side the bread will fall on or our chances of being on time to the office, we find pretty soon that events follow natural laws and there is no outside force interfering in them.

Again, it might be said that the Force had decreed these laws at the beginning of the world and ensured that everything followed them, and thus brought about the universe that it desired. Once the world was started off in a particular way, the laws ensured that it would evolve only in this particular way, and thus all events that have occurred and are going to occur have already been predetermined right from the start of the world at the big bang.

The final point that contradicts all such rigid determinism is that of quantum physics. Quantum physics has shown that there is no absolute determinism in the world of subatomic events. For any given event, we can only predict the range of probable results, out of which any particular result may occur. If this ambiguity is a part of the quantum world, it means that it is also a part of our "everyday world," the macroscopic world, and it is only because we do not consider these minute deviations when we consider the events in our world that we see a rigidly deterministic world. Thus quantum physics rules out any such determinism; even if the laws were decreed at the beginning, each event had many outcomes, and there could have been an infinite number of final outcomes. It was purely out of random chance that the particular series of outcomes that resulted in our specific world happened to occur.

Such a concept of a rigid fate, which binds us all from the beginning to the end, has given rise to intriguing aspects of human behavior such as the belief in astrology and other predictive arts. Astrology is based on the belief that the whole universe moves in a predetermined cycle. All individual cycles (the microcosm) are related and a part of this all-encompassing cycle (the macrocosm). Hence, by studying the position of the stars at the point of birth, we can determine the point at which our microcosmic cycle "enters" or becomes a part of this macrocosmic cycle, and then at any particular time determine where our "microcosmic" cycle stands in relation to the "macrocosmic" cycle as it is being dragged along with it. We can thus understand the position of our life, as some points in the relationship between the macrocosm and the microcosm are said to be inimical and some beneficial.

Other predictive methods also depend on similar logic. If all events in the world were interconnected, then the result of even the smallest event would be directly connected to the course of our life. Thus an apparently random event would not be random, but would ultimately be connected to the rest of our life. So it is certainly possible that the card we draw from a pack or the fortune cookie drawn for us by a parrot is predictive of other things. Similarly, the lines on our hand or the numbers in our name are also connected to the course of our life. By a long process of studying such events and their association with humans, practitioners of predictive arts like these claim that they have been able to discover the relationship between random events and aspects of human lives.

The argument against this is the same as that which was already given: that randomness is an inbuilt part of the universe, and it does not follow a strictly predetermined course. Each event could have a number of potential subsequent events, and so there is no rigid line of cause and effect. Grand views of macrocosm and microcosm cannot stand against a mathematical analysis of events.

Another similar question regarding our own actions is that of fate versus will. This is an age-old argument between two viewpoints, one that maintains that our actions are rigidly controlled by outside forces so that everything we do or think is predetermined by the circumstances around us, and one that upholds that we have a free will to do the things that we want to do.

The main point about this argument is whether we have any choice in our actions. The modern argument for fate or determinism is that we are rigidly controlled by the events in our development, our genes plus our environment, in such a way that there is no freedom of choice in our actions. This would mean that at every event in life, our course of action is already dictated by our past, so that if we have a super-intelligent being who knew all our genes and the events in our life, he would be able to predict exactly what we would do in a given circumstance.

The important point to consider in this argument is that we are learning machines. Our capacity to learn means that we are able to take in data from our environment and change our behavioral patterns or "programs" accordingly—that is, change our way of deciding and thinking. We retain our learning capacity throughout our lives, which means that we are continually changing and hence "reprogramming" ourselves. For example, if we learn to play the violin, we are quite obviously changing our behavior because we have acquired a new behavior. In addition, such learning will affect what we do in our lives in new ways, so that we follow music more and try to listen to it more often and so on.

The ability to learn by itself indicates that we have decision-making abilities, because during the process of learning we have to continuously mold our behavior to weed out mistakes and make corrections. Each time we learn something, our behavioral patterns change in many ways, and since we are learning or "unlearning" things at every moment, our patterns of behavior cannot be rigidly bound. Each time our behavior changes, we are again exposed to new things to learn or not to learn. The presence of our capacity to learn indicates that we *do* have free will.

Among all species, the learning capacity is the highest in humans; hence it is humans whose "will" is the "freest," so to say. The behavior of lower animals is more and more automatic, as they do not change their behavioral patterns easily, and in the lowest, there is no change at all. This capacity to change our behavior rapidly has ensured our survival and this has been the greatest advantage of our species. Hence our adaptability shows us that we are not governed by a strict fate and we retain the capacity to change ourselves all the time: we have a free will.

A similar argument is made by proponents of major religions: God controls all our actions and so we do not have any free will. This can be refuted in the same way: if we have the capacity to learn, it means that God has to allow us freedom of choice in our actions so that we can learn, and so God loses his rigid control over us.

The ability to learn has given rise to the concept of "memes." Memes might be called a unit of learning. The path of an elephant herd to a watering hole is a meme for an elephant and is transmitted from one to the other. The elephants holding the highest number of such memes become the leaders, as they have the highest survival capability.

Memes are by far the most highly developed in humans. It is believed that this explosion in human memes was because of the development of speech and language, which gave us the ability to transmit more and more complex memes much more widely. Evolution based on genes is a slow and unsure process. The further evolution of humankind will be through the progress of our memes. While this is completely different from genetic evolution in that it is not "physical," it will be as vital in terms of increasing our ability to dominate our environment and hence our ability to survive as we struggle to conquer in ever-newer environments, such as outer space.

Much of the dominance of humans over other animals is in fact due to our memes and not our genes. Groups of people living in a primitive state are cut off from this knowledge pool, and they have little advantage over animals in their domination of the environment. They have access to only their own isolated meme pools. But when meme pools of different groups merge, forming a larger pool, the ability to dominate increases greatly. As the knowledge of larger and larger groups of humans is shared, our strength will also increase accordingly.

In this context the Information Age carries a great significance for our future. New tools of communication such as telephones and the Internet have added a whole new dimension to the transmission of memes, and they are probably as important a milestone in human progress as the development of speech. It will mean an explosion in our evolution and our ability to respond to our environment.

Those who have known the vital force of the vital force, the eye of the eye, the ear of the ear, and the mind of the mind, have realized the ancient primordial Brahman.
    —Brihadaranyaka Upanishad IV.iv.18

Another question that arises is that of our individuality. Because our individual feelings and thoughts are private, we can never know another person's mind. We may ask whether other people are really like us: do they see the same thing inside their heads as we do when we see a red color, for instance? Do they feel the same thing as us when we feel angry or happy? Our daily interactions of course are built on an assumption that we share the same feelings, but it seems difficult to prove logically.

Here too evolutionary theory has helped in solving this old philosophical quandary. By seeing ourselves as products of an evolutionary process, we can see that no person is an isolated individual. We are all part of a common inheritance, and in fact we are part of the entire chain of life. All our physical and mental processes are part of a common chain of development.

During evolution, each species occupied its own specific niche. Those species would survive best that understood their environment the most. Hence evolution ensured that benefits were assigned to the power of recognizing the environment and adapting to it. This ensured the development of the senses in the earliest species, and these senses gradually became more and more refined. Vision, for example, would begin with some species developing light-sensitive sensors, which in time gradually developed into the eye.

The earliest species to develop color vision would begin by having light-sensitive sensors, which were triggered by only a particular narrow band of light. When such a creature came before the color red, for example, its eye would react to it and the brain would recognize it. This sensation of seeing red and also other colors would give it evolutionary advantages, and color vision would be transmitted down the line. That's why our vision and the sensations we gather with our eyes are not an individual experience, but something we share in common with all members of our species—and, in fact, with a very large number of other species. We have inherited the same organ of vision and the "hardware" in the brain connected with it from older species. Hence when we see the color red, we can be quite certain that we are having the same experience in our mind that would be had by all other humans and in fact by all animals too.

Besides the senses, the species also acquired an understanding of such concepts as time and distance in order to survive. They would acquire such concepts as would be best suited for their survival. The concept of time for a fruit fly, which lives its entire life cycle within one week, will be different from that of humans. So too the concept of distance would be different for an ant. But within the same species the same basic concept for time and distance would be inherited and shared. Emotions like anger, fear, and joy would also be held in common. Hence evolution ensures that our basic concepts of life are the same. We can be sure that the emotions we feel, the basic fundamentals of our thinking, and the way we learn and make decisions are the same for all of us. As we have a common mental structure, we are able to develop a common language and understand each other.

Babies coming into the world have these basic concepts hardwired in their brains. They also have the capacity to learn, which ultimately translates into freedom of will, hardwired in their brains. Through their senses, they gradually acquire knowledge of their new and external world and develop increasingly complicated ideas.

The basic numerical ability to distinguish between one or many objects is a part of this mental ability. Mathematics is also only a language, with the numbers and other signs being equivalent to words; we describe a particular aspect of the world using these words. As mathematics evolved, it developed more and more complex ways of describing the world. All of these shared abilities assure us that there is a common base to our knowledge and senses.

The concept of evolution in epistemology provides us with a basis to understand our knowledge and experience and how we can relate them to those of others. With this advance, human knowledge and the process of learning has now shed much of its mystery and seeming paradoxes.

> *Let my vital force now attain the all-pervading immortal air;*
> *and now let this body be reduced to ashes. Om, my mind,*
> *remember—remember all that has been done. O mind,*
> *remember all that has been done.*
>
> —Isa Upanishad XVII

Despite all this progress in understanding philosophy, two fundamental mysteries remain unanswered: life and death. The difficulty in defining life, its mechanics and metaphysics, has been subject to intense speculation through the ages. In general, a living organism may be called that which *reacts* to its environment. A nonliving object such as a rock is only *acted* upon by its environment. Something such as a storm is also acted upon by its environment, which becomes stronger when its environment is energy rich and weaker otherwise. A candle or a piece of wood has stored-up energy; when the environment stimulates it with fire, it quickly and automatically disperses the energy through flames.

But a living body is able to *react* to the environment in that it can sense its environment, judge whether it is harmful or beneficial, and accordingly change itself in some way, or change its behavior. An amoeba will move away from extreme hot or cold environments and try to move towards equilibrium. It will also move towards energy-rich environments, that is, environments containing food. Even a virus reacts to its environment: when it finds a suitable host, it changes from its dormant state and begins multiplying. Another characteristic of a living body is, of course, that it multiplies, producing offspring similar to it. Hence a living body is never found alone but in a species.

This ability to sense and react to the environment suggests a strange power, a supernatural power. Religions throughout the ages have made a clear distinction between living and nonliving things, believing God, the supreme supernatural being, to have granted this power. But as we have seen, medical knowledge has already advanced to a stage where we do not need to conceive of any supernatural entity to account for life or consciousness. The presence of the soul is contradicted not only by modern scientific and biological knowledge, but also by logical reasoning and philosophical understanding.

Sometimes such a widespread belief in, say, the soul or God

among many different peoples gives rise to the idea that since these ideas are universal, there must be something behind it and these ideas must be true. The universality of an idea, however, cannot be accepted as a basis for believing in it. People throughout the centuries and across all cultures have believed that the earth is flat, yet this does not mean it is true. So also beliefs in things like spirits and ghosts are also universal.

When confronted with a puzzle, the nature of thinking being similar, people usually tend to arrive at similar solutions. This need not make a solution appear true. Even our instinctive knowledge or intuition need not be true. Our innate knowledge of time is that it is a constant, but relativity proves both theoretically and practically that there is no fixed time, which is counterintuitive. Yet this is true and cannot be denied.

The main problem with understanding life is understanding consciousness—our own consciousness. It is difficult to define consciousness logically, but in simple terms, consciousness can be considered to be awareness, awareness of the self and of the external environment. Defined in this way, life itself is consciousness, and hence consciousness can be said to be present in every living body. An amoeba is able to analyze its environment and then react appropriately by moving away or toward the stimuli for its survival. This too is consciousness of some sort.

The ability of a virus to change its state and multiply in a suitable environment or change into a dormant state when it is in a hostile environment also shows an ability to sense the environment and react to it. Hence this too is consciousness in its most primitive form. It signifies that the organism is aware of both the environment and itself, though of course this awareness is in its most rudimentary state. Even in the highest of the animals, their awareness, both of the self and of the external environment, is very much lower than that of humans.

In man, both self-awareness and the ability to understand the external environment are seen in its highest form. Our consciousness is difficult to explain in terms of physical and chemical reactions, and the soul is an easy explanation.

Besides the physiological difficulties, another problem in assuming a supernatural basis of consciousness, such as the soul, is deciding where to draw this line. Viruses, as we know, can react to the environment, and so can be said to have consciousness. But it is difficult to assume a soul for the virus, which is nothing more than a soup of chemicals. Amoeba and other single-celled organisms are much more like what we understand as living organisms, actively searching and preying on their food, and also moving about. But it still seems odd, to say the least, to talk about the soul of an amoeba. But all living beings proceed gradually up the scale, from single-celled organisms to multi-cellular ones, and finally further up the scale to humankind. There is no place where there is a sudden change in the scale to the extent that we can affirm that the soul is present from here.

Religions were often forced to draw the line arbitrarily. In India, the Buddhists drew the line at trees, and declared that unmoving, living objects like trees did not have a soul. The arbitrariness of this view drew sharp criticism, and there were long and heated arguments by their opponents on this view. Perhaps it was just as well that amoebae and viruses had not yet been discovered!

Another place to draw the line, which suggested itself naturally, was between humans and all other living beings. This is because we are self-aware and we feel a fundamental difference with other species.

Do we say the soul is present only in human beings? Then we would be saying that consciousness is present only in humans as only the soul is supposed to have consciousness. That would be ridiculous, as certainly other animals are not unconscious. On the other hand, if consciousness is produced without a soul in animals, then there is no need to posit it for humans. We can, of course, also say that only human consciousness is true consciousness, because it is fundamentally higher than animal consciousness and hence only humans have souls. Animal consciousness, being of a lower order, could be produced by their brains alone.

This would mean two different types of consciousness, one in humans brought about by a soul, and one in all other species of animals that is brought about by the brain alone. However, such a position contradicts all known science. It contradicts evolution, as man is clearly shown to be an animal and descended from other animals. There is no place for a sudden jump in which human consciousness changes completely from other animals. It contradicts anatomy and physiology, as the brain of other animals like the chimpanzee is shown to be not fundamentally different from humans; hence their consciousness also cannot be fundamentally different from humans. Chimpanzees cannot have a completely different mechanism from humans for their "untrue" consciousness. All this would contradict positing a soul only for humans. It is far more coherent to say that our individual consciousness is produced by our bodies, or rather by our brains, and there is no supernatural entity like the soul as its basis.

A further problem with theorizing the existence of something like the soul lies in defining how it interacts with the body. Conscious impulses such as sensations are undoubtedly a part of the body, because it is when odors assail us or a pin pricks us that we get these sensations. But if the soul is an independent, nonmaterial entity in the body, how do these impulses reach the soul? It means that the soul has to be connected with the body at some stage. Such a connection would also be required when our consciousness—that is, our soul—directs the movements of the body. But where would the soul connect with the body? Certainly there is no evidence of any such non-material thing connecting with the body anywhere. Such theories of the soul contradict all known scientific knowledge, and also contradict logic and reason, being based purely on doctrinal definitions.

Recent developments in understanding the brain are increasingly showing us that there is no need to assume a supernatural basis for consciousness. It is now universally accepted in medical science that our consciousness is based on the hum of electro-physical interactions in the brain. Diseases of the "consciousness," our mind, are regularly dealt with and treated effectively on this basis. Drugs like antidepressants are taken for depression, and by doing so we are in fact changing the state of our consciousness by altering the chemical balance in the brain. In fact, this has been done throughout the centuries without accepting its implications.

In general, we assume our emotions to be the most integral and sacred part of our "I-ness." We would like to believe them to be a part of the soul and do not want to believe them to be connected with chemicals. Yet we have always used chemical substances to change our emotions, as when we take marijuana or alcohol. If we can accept that something so vital as our emotions are based on chemical reactions, there seems little difficulty in accepting that the rest of our "I-ness" is also based on chemical reactions. Medicines can also alter the pattern of our thoughts, such as suicidal thoughts, and alter behavior. All these show that our individual consciousness, our "I-ness," is a product of the brain, and hence can be altered by altering the material constituents of the brain.

The brain has billions of nerve cells, which are interconnected and organized for different functions in much the same way as the rest of the body. There are specialized areas for movement (sensations, speech, memories, etc.). Very little is known today of how feelings and emotions are generated, or even how memories are stored. But it is known from surgical experiments that stimulation of certain areas will revive old memories with all their attendant emotions. The brain in some way is clearly able to store emotions, because we can "sense" them again when we remember them, and so it is quite logical that through its connections it should be able to generate emotions as well. Some areas of the brain, such as the speech learning area, are also specially equipped for learning. If it is not stimulated before the age of six, the child is unable to learn speech, so the learning capacity too is a special function of the brain.

Thus, although believing our consciousness is produced by the brain alone is difficult, there seems to be no other alternative. There is as yet a great deal to understand about consciousness. But the only thing that it appears we can be sure of is that there is no need to postulate an "out-of-nature" supernatural entity as an explanation.

> *Gargya said, "This being who identifies himself with the shadow, I meditate upon him as Brahman."*
> *Ajatashatru said, "Please don't talk about him. I meditate upon him as death."*
> —Brihadaranyaka Upanishad II.i.12

Along with consciousness, the other characteristic of life is death. Life and death are like two sides of a coin, coexisting and defining each other. There has been perhaps more philosophical speculation on death than there has been on life. Death is the ultimate mystery. It is almost certain that no matter how advanced we become, we will never be able to get an answer. Religions in fact depend more on death than life to draw in their followers by promising a life after death.

Why does death happen? It is not that all living organisms must die. The smallest organisms, the single-celled ones, do not die. In single-celled organisms, the same cell necessarily has to do all the functions like food gathering, digestion, and excretion. Each cell is a complete and self-contained organism. Perhaps because of their independent functioning, they are able to continue their lives without any end, although they can be killed by accident.

In multi-celled organisms there are different cells for each function, with some cells collecting food while others digest it and still others carrying out excretion. Each cell is specialized and can carry out only its own function, depending on others for the rest. Because of this specialization, it is probable that the cells are not able to function in totality, and as their excretion and fault-correcting mechanisms are not in full play, toxins and defects gather in the cell with time. Hence multi-celled organisms have to die after some time. This is one theory of death.

This process of death by toxification would have meant a slow uphill course until the organism acquired full maturity and then another gradual downhill one until its death. But in evolution, mathematically an organism would be able to produce a greater number of offspring if it had a burst of a highly active reproductive stage, even if that meant its downhill course was far sharper.

The advantage of a short but potent burst of reproductive ability pushed organisms toward having a peak of youth, though it also meant a quicker fall into the degeneration of old age and death. In essence, we have old age because we have youth. Eventually, this reproductive advantage led all organisms to a predetermined lifecycle of adolescence, youth, and old age, terminating in death.

Death is a problem that will always haunt us. In the Mahabharata, Yudhisthir, on being asked to name the most incomprehensible fact in the world, says that it is that humans, knowing they are going to die, are yet able to carry on their normal life without apparently worrying about it much. As Nobel laureate and scientist Richard Feynman (1918–1988) put it, if immortal aliens came to Earth and were confronted with the knowledge that death is inevitable for humans, they would never be able to understand how we could go on living with this burden.

We do it with a mixture of stoicism and calm indifference, regarding death as a natural and inevitable event. Despite our knowledge that we will someday die, we do not acknowledge death on a daily basis and cannot actually conceive of a time when we will no longer exist. The fact that death is inevitable for everyone is also a great source of satisfaction. Even so, death haunts us in our songs, poetry, music, and day-to-day thoughts and conversations.

It is from this daily haunting that religions draw their main strength. All religions are based primarily on making death palatable to us, and usually more time is spent on this than on understanding life. Death is made palatable in a variety of ways, most commonly by promising us a life after death. A further life is promised in heaven, which will be immortal and include all the good things that we didn't get the first time. Death then becomes a nonevent, merely the beginning of a better life. Of course all this comes only for believers; the rest get such a terrible time in hell that they are soon wishing for a second death.

Beliefs about death, although differing in each religion, are broadly similar and can be classified into three groups depending on the degree of merger into the final truth. This is determined by the way humans are defined in relation to God, or the final truth, in that philosophy.

The most common idea that we have about religious beliefs on death is the simple dualistic belief. In dualism, the soul of a person is considered to be a separate entity from God, and also immortal. When the person dies, or the vessel breaks, the soul is set free. From this point, what happens next is mere speculation. All dualistic views, in Christianity, Islam, and dualistic Hinduism, are more or less similar, with individual takes on the same basic principle.

In the somewhat fantastical accounts of simple dualism, once people die, their souls are transported to a nether space, where they are put to judgment. The people then apparently come up before God in a way that is rather similar to a court scene. The final outcome is that the souls gets judged and sent to heaven if they are found clean, or to hell if not. Hereafter, the souls remain finally immortal, with no further death or judgments, and enjoy all kinds of amusements or suffer tortures, as the case may be, throughout eternity.

A good number of arguments can be made against nearly all the points in such a fanciful speculation. The confounding factors of moral judgments, such as genetic or environmental issues, seem to cut no ice with God, who has to make simple and rigid decisions. The laws imposed on us according to the doctrines are also quite strict, and it appears that hardly anyone would get past them and into heaven, with rules related to lying, lust, and greed being probably the most flouted. Even the scare of going to hell doesn't seem to give us the strength to control these risks to our immortal lives.

Such simple-minded tales seem to have the sole aim of keeping a raised whip over the followers of religions to ensure they stick to it, but such tales are not really needed. Neither Hinduism nor Christianity, Islam, or any other successful religion would have attracted followers based solely on such mythology. It is because they have much more to offer that they have achieved their greatness.

Another way of understanding death is the theory of reincarnation in Hinduism and Buddhism. In dualism the soul remains eternally separate from God in heaven or hell, but here, the soul ultimately becomes a part of the absolute. Before that it has to undergo multiple births in numerous bodies until it succeeds in living a perfect life.

In reincarnation, the soul is believed to be the living part of the body, the driver in the car, and can exist independently of the body. In fact, here the soul is the real person and the body a mere appendage. The reincarnation theory is conjoined with the theory of Karma. When the soul takes birth in a body, it acquires all the Karma that is done by that person in his or her life, with good deeds and bad deeds being added up against each other. Death is envisioned as a death of the body only; the Bhagavad Gita describes it as a change of clothes for the soul. People who have more bad deeds in their book than good have to take rebirth as a lower form of life, while those with better records get a higher life. The thought at the point of death, which is determined by the course of the whole life, is said to play the determining effect—"together with whatever thought he had at the time of death, he becomes merged into prana," according to the Prasna Upanishad.

Because of this belief, Mahatma Gandhi, whose dying words were "Hei Ram," the name of the Lord, earned even greater reverence in India and confirmation of his saintly status through his death. When people finally overtake bad Karma and achieve perfection in life, they get *mukti*. There are no more rebirths for them and they merge into the absolute. The nature of the merging differs depending on the religious sect. In Hinduism, the individual soul is said to merge with Brahman, while in Buddhism, it merges into nothingness, or *shunya*. In some qualified monistic doctrines, it is believed that the soul retains a vestige of personality, and so the merger is not complete.

This system has the advantage that it promises *mukti*, a final merging of the soul into the absolute, but it suffers from the same basic defect as dualism. There seems to be no logic whatsoever to the theory. It is another tale laid down by scriptural doctrines with no practical or logical arguments in its support. Other defects, like the difficulty of moral judgments and how and where this law of Karma came from, are also there. How exactly the soul enters into the human body and at what point is also not easily explained.

The Upanishads give an intriguing explanation for this. At death, the soul goes into the sky. There it mixes with rain and falls down. Then, if it is at the appropriate stage, it enters into the crops and becomes a grain of rice. It is eaten by a man and enters into his semen where it finally enters a human body when the man impregnates a woman! All kinds of difficulties are associated with the theory of reincarnation, with questions such as whether a worm, or to be more modern, an amoeba or virus, has a soul. If a particularly bad man were to end up in an amoeba, it seems he would have met a dead end, because it seems almost impossible for an amoeba to do enough good deeds to ascend up the scale! These explanations are as unsatisfactory as others, and add more to the mystery of death.

The final belief is that of Advaita. Here there is no true death because there is no true reality. All manifestations are unreal and limitations of Brahman; therefore, when the individual dies, what dies is the unreal part of him or her. The true part is released from all limitations and Brahman shines through. This idea of death is a part of the metaphysical beliefs of Advaita.

> *From the dark I wish to attain the delightful. Having shaken off sin, like a horse shaking its hair, I shall attain the uncreated world of Brahman after leaving this body and become successful.*
> *I shall attain.*
>
> —Chandogya Upanishad VIII.xiii.1

To understand ourselves, we need to understand not just death, but life and all its various mysteries. We need to develop a philosophy to explain the universe and our role in it. Countless philosophies have been defined by trying to find a perfect solution to this mystery of existence. The branch of philosophy involved in trying to understand existence is called metaphysics. With time, the different metaphysical positions have become refined and exhaustive, with each system having its own adherents and strong and weak points.

The most common way to explain our existence is to define a force, which is outside the universe. This force is not limited by the universe, and, hence, can create and control it. Such a force, although defined in various ways by each religion, is called God. The main positions regarding the nature of God may be defined as dualism, qualified monism, and monism. Atheism, agnosticism, and nihilism are viewpoints that have arisen from a variety of stands on these positions.

Nihilism is the position that denies the world, and may be of different types, such as moral nihilism or political nihilism. In metaphysical nihilism, the *existence* of the world itself is denied. Nothing exists, says the nihilist, and all the world is a mere dream, which will disappear as soon as we realize this. Such pure nihilism is rather difficult to swallow, but its strength lies in the fierce and crippling attacks it can launch against attempts by other creeds to show that something *does* exist.

Atheism, as it is commonly understood, means a belief that there is no God. However, this is not an exact definition, because before we can say that there is no God, we have to first define God. An atheist may willingly proclaim his disbelief of a creative and grand old figure, like the Gods of most religions, but the absolute as defined in Advaitism and Buddhism is not such a figure, and many who feel they are atheists might accept such logic. A strong atheistic statement that there is no God also shows a belief. A true atheist should by definition have no "belief." Hence, it would be better to say that atheists are those who do not believe in any creed. They can define their belief only in relation to that of others. A true atheist is one who does not accept any belief; he would say that each belief is wrong and, hence, that he does not believe in it.

The position of an agnostic is also related to other creeds, rather than being a creed of its own. Agnostics maintain that because no religious creed can be scientifically proven, the truth of any creed, along with the existence of God, is essentially unknowable. Again, the question arises as to what exactly *it* is that cannot be known.

Agnostics may not concern themselves with the problem of defining God, but with immediate knowledge of the world, which is certain. They do not involve themselves in endless speculation over a matter that they feel can never be resolved. Agnosticism, like atheism, is best defined against other creeds, by saying that the agnostic does not take interest in any creed because it cannot be either proved or disproved by the scientific method.

To each creed that arises, the atheist will say, "I do not believe because you are wrong." The agnostic will say, "I do not believe because your creed can neither be proved nor disproved." Modern scientific thought usually veers to one of these two positions; however, the majority of people in the world believe in one of a variety of creeds. The definitions of God in different creeds are considered to be of three types in Hindu philosophy: dualism, qualified monism, and absolute monism.

Monism is to be differentiated from *monotheism*. Monotheism is the concept that there is one God, and is opposed to polytheism, which is the belief in many gods or supernatural forces. Monotheism and polytheism are both creeds of dualism because they accept the reality of two distinct entities, namely the world and God or gods. On the other hand, in monism there is only *one* reality. All things that exist are but different manifestations of a single entity; all things are One.

In dualism, God is defined as a supernatural force who, by His will, creates us all and rules over us. The God of dualism is a being entirely separate from the world. He exists prior to the world and creates it for a definite purpose. He also creates humans and everything else in this world and rules over it all. The God of dualism is invariably a personal God who is involved with humans in creating, ruling, and, finally, judging them.

Such is the God of most religions, including the most common strains of Christianity, Islam, Judaism, and dualistic Hinduism. The gods are often anthropomorphic, and conceived of in terms of a particular human appearance, as in the examples of Jesus or Krishna. In Islam, Allah is not anthropomorphic, as he is thought to be inconceivable. However, Allah is a personal God because he is involved with human activity. It is also important to note that the rise of male patriarchy supported the conception of most personal gods as male. Greeks, Egyptians, and early Romans did have female personal gods, but in present-day religion, female gods are seen mainly in Hinduism, most notably in Tantric sects, where the female is considered to be all-powerful.

In dualism, humans and God are considered to be on two different levels. There is no junction between them and man is not a part of God in any sense. Therefore, in dualism humans cannot touch God, and the nearest that we can come is to have a vision of the Almighty.

In qualified monism, humans are considered to originate from God. The god of qualified monism is also a personal god with will. He creates the world and all humans, but he creates it out of his own substance. Thus, qualified monism does not recognize the dualistic idea that there is a fundamental difference between the nature of humans and the nature of God. Instead, qualified monists believe that there is a divine spark in all humans and in all parts of the world. In such a philosophy, everyone is a part of the Lord. We are a part and God is the whole.

The god of qualified monism is usually not an anthropomorphic god, as he is considered to be formless, but he is still a personal god because he interacts with humans, has will, and creates humans due to his will. He also rules over them all and judges them. In this belief system, humans have a higher status than in dualism, as they are a part of God, and therefore, potentially divine. In qualified monism, humans can touch and feel God within themselves. All humans have the spark of divinity. God is to be looked for not in the heavens, but within us.

Monism is the philosophy of the absolute. In monism, the world and all its constituents are different manifestations of a single reality. This absolute reality is called Brahman in Hinduism. Everything that exists is a different form of this entity, and there is nothing in the world that is not Brahman. All that we see, hear, taste, touch, smell, think, and feel is Brahman. All parts of us are Brahman, including our individual consciousness. There is no power outside the universe that can control Brahman or rule over it.

Philosophical speculation through the ages has developed a very large number of positions on varying subjects. With such a volume of thought, it is almost impossible to come to a definite solution to any particular issue; however, reason demands that we should accept the philosophical system or religion that best aligns with scientific knowledge. The rigorous logic of Advaitism and Buddhism enables these philosophies to stand up to modern scientific thought and embrace it. Much about the world remains unknown today, and the quest for human knowledge will doubtless continue to shed new light on these issues.

Advaita Theory

*It rested set upon the Unborn's navel, that One wherein
    abide all things existing.
Ye will not find Him who produced these creatures;
    another thing hath risen up among you.
Enwrapt in misty cloud, with lips that stammer,
Ye hymn-chanters wander and are discontented.*

—Rig Veda, 10.82

Advaita is the Sanskrit term for non-duality (from *dvaita*, meaning duality). The philosophy of Advaita declares that there is only one reality. There is no second. All that exists is one. Advaitism is derived from the writings of the Upanishads (also known as Vedanta), and it is the most rigorous of the three Vedantic schools (dualistic, qualified monistic, and monistic).

An Advaitic inquiry into the nature of things begins with two basic questions concerning two kinds of knowledge: knowledge about the self—that is, ourselves—and knowledge about the world. It is these questions that are defined and their answers that are sought in the Upanishads.

The Katha Upanishad tells the story of a young prince named Nachiketas who seeks to increase his knowledge about the self. At the tale's outset, Nachiketas has been banished by his father in a fit of rage, and is sent to wait on Yama, the Hindu god of death. When he arrives at Yama's palace, the gate is locked and he must wait outside for three days and three nights. On the fourth day, Yama finally appears and grants Nachiketas three boons, one for each day he waited. For his third, final, and most important boon, Nachiketas asks Yama a question. "Consequent on the death of a person, a doubt arises when some say 'it exists' while some say 'it does not exist,'" he says. "What is the reality?"

This is the question about a person's inner awareness and knowledge of the self. Yama's answer symbolizes the transfer of knowledge about the self from the gods to mankind. Yama tells Nachiketas that only those things that are unreal and are compounds can die. For that which is true, there can be no death. As Yama rules death, he alone can distinguish that which is undying from that which is mortal. The remainder of the Katha Upanishad records the rest of Yama's answer to this question.

The Mundaka Upanishad addresses the second question, regarding our knowledge of the external environment and objects that surround us. In the Mundaka Upanishad, it is asked, "Which is that thing, which having been known, all this becomes known?" Here, the effort is to go from the particular to the general. To know the composition of the earth, for example, we need not study the whole of the earth. By collecting and studying a lump of the earth, we can get to know about the whole. This, of course, implicitly states that knowledge can be generalized—that is, that by studying a lump, we can generalize our findings and apply them to the earth as a whole. The Upanishad asks whether or not this is true. In other words, "Is there something by knowing which all this can be known?"

The seers, or *rishis*, of the Upanishads were guided by a desire to know and understand the world. They sought to know the outer world, the world of phenomena, and the inner world, the world of the "self." The seers were not guided by experimental science in their quest, but relied on logic and the intuition gathered by meditation. Information gathered by meditation was given primacy, but such findings became acceptable only when they rested on a bedrock of correct logic.

The Upanishadic seers were dissatisfied with the commonsense view of the world, in which we accept our first impressions as truth. They saw that this phenomenal world was not a sufficient explanation in itself, and it did not hold up to investigation when probed more thoroughly. The sages declared that our everyday world was not the sole truth, and that existence had two levels—the phenomenal plane, or the plane of our daily existence, and the absolute plane, the plane of Brahman, the god of the Upanishads.

The Upanishadic declaration of an absolute plane was interpreted by the three schools of Vedanta in various ways, leading to three very different theories of the true nature of the world and God. The dualistic school said that both the world and Brahman are equally real, and the two are fundamentally different from each other. The qualified monists also accepted both the world and Brahman as equally real, but they said that the world is a form of God, created by God out of his own substance, so it too, is of a divine nature. The most far-reaching interpretation is that of the Advaitists, who declared that the only true existence is that of Brahman. For them, the phenomenal world was untrue and existence was relative.

The Advaitic interpretation, although the most esoteric, was also the most logical, and other schools of thought accepted it as such. A popular argument against Advaita was that it appealed only to the mind, and not to the heart. With beliefs based so firmly on reason, Advaita was missing the loving and supportive personal god so familiar to most believers.

Advaita based its teachings on the findings of the Upanishadic sages during meditation, and follows up their findings with a rigid application of logic and reason, which allows no weakness or falsity. In this way they built up a worldview that does not depend on any doctrine for support, and which is able to explain the facts of the world in a logical, self-contained, and somewhat astounding form.

The Upanishads and Advaitism analyze the world from a realistic metaphysical viewpoint. Prior to any metaphysical speculation, it accepts the trio of thinker, thought, and the thing thought of as existing on the same plane of reality. Thus, the thinker, the subject, and the object lie on the same plane of existence and have equally and antecedently the same level of reality. Starting from this realistic viewpoint, the rishis then set about to understand the "reality" of both the outside world and the inner one.

When we examine the phenomena of the world logically, each phenomenon is eventually found to be contradictory to logic, and no basis for its real existence can be found. There is no universal or absolute reality in anything that we see around us. The old paradox of determining whether time and space is finite or infinite is well known. Space is meaningless unless an object is present in it. Likewise, an object cannot exist without space. Hence, both are untrue in themselves; they can only exist together. If they are two different things, then they should be able to exist separately. On the other hand, they cannot be the same thing, either, for they have contrary natures.

The problem with defining time is similar. We cannot determine what that moment is that we call the present. We find, if we look closely, that there is not a single, standing, unmoving moment that we can call the present. On the other hand, if we assume that the present is just the interface where the future changes into the past, then we also assume that there are blocks of future and past time, which is as difficult to understand and prove as a block of time called the present. Also, at the interface, both the future and the past must exist simultaneously where they touch, which cannot be possible.

Such arguments show that we cannot understand anything of the nature of time or space. Yet time and space are inherent in the nature of all phenomena, and if they are contradictory, then all phenomena must be contradictory.

The ancient seers meditated on objects and tried to find out the basis of their reality. They discovered that no such basis could be found in any object in the universe. All things in the universe are constantly changing. Matter and energy are, as it were, constantly flowing from one whirlpool of an object to another. It is to these temporary whirlpools that we give names, and which we consider as being some existing "thing." Even our bodies are constantly changing. It is calculated that all the cells that make up our bodies are changed and renewed every seven years. Literally, we are not now the people that we were seven years ago.

If a thing is constantly changing, it cannot be considered absolutely real. Its reality will be relative, existing only for a temporary period. It will depend on the observer of that moment for its reality. Since these conditions are true for all things in the phenomenal world, it must be true that nothing in this world has a permanent or absolute reality.

The reality of the world is only something that is defined by our senses—or, rather, by our interpretation of sensory information. For example, if we take a thing such as a table, it seems very solid and real to us. The table is defined by all its "qualities," or properties (solidity, shape, color, etc.). All of these qualities may seem real, but we know from science that, in fact, the table is only a collection of molecules, and the vast part of it, between the molecules, is empty space. Even a molecule is composed of mostly empty space; actual matter is a very small fraction of its makeup.

Molecules and atoms are not well-defined "masses" at all, but a conglomeration of fuzzy forces. When we "see" a table or "touch" it, we depend on our minds to interpret the way that light affects our eyes, and the way that the molecules of our fingers react with the molecules of the table. The mind's interpretation of sensory input gives only an approximate view. As a result, we experience a "solid" table, and not the true reality of an amorphous mass of space and ill-defined forces.

Similarly, when Upanishadic seers meditated on and applied logic to other interrelations within the world, such as the law of cause and effect, they found the relationships to be contradictory—each one gave rise to paradoxes. With such contradictions as a premise, Advaitists argued against the idea that any object has a true form, against the existence of objects in time and space, and against change. Virtually all ideas that we have of the world were declared false.

It is these factors—time, space, matter-energy, cause-effect, and so forth—that give definition to the world and allow us to accept it as a reality. If these are contradictory, then the idea of a well-defined *real* world is wrong, and this world, our everyday world, does not exist as the place we normally perceive. Instead, the world must be ill-defined and non-deterministic. Advaita declares that the world is illusory. Here, Illusion does not mean that the world does not exist, but that we perceive this amorphous and undefined world as a well-defined, concrete reality.

Such a conclusion, as was to be expected, was heavily criticized even in ancient India, and the Advaitic philosophy was sometimes considered a mere word game, using logic to arrive at an absurd conclusion. In the past, other religious leaders and philosophers generally viewed Advaita in the same way when they came up against it for the first time. But whatever criticisms Advaitia may have been subject to in the past, its ideas are surprisingly similar to many in contemporary science today.

Einstein's theory of relativity has demonstrated that definitions of time and space are relative to observation. There is no such thing as fixed time and space, permanent object size, or even stable mass. Our habitual perception of the world works relatively— it works for the everyday world, but is not actually true. Advaitic philosophers concluded the same thing thousands of years ago through the application of logic.

Quantum physics has been the most important development in proving the contentions of Advaitism through the study of phenomena. Like Advaitic philosophers, contemporary physicists declare that the quantum world does not truly possess "classical" Newtonian properties. In fact, our world is ill-defined, and lacks any absolute reality. At first, convincing the world to accept quantum physics proved as difficult as convincing the world to accept Advaitism, but its conclusions are inescapable, and the "fuzzy" reality of the world is something that we all have to learn to live with. Thus, modern science has finally proven the contention of Advaita, and also of Buddhism, that the world has only an ill-defined, or illusory, reality, and these two religious traditions are today the only ones consistent with our present knowledge of the world.

Through meditation, Advaitic scholars arrived at another important conclusion. It is not just the outer world that lacks an absolute reality, but the inner world, including individual consciousness. During meditation, Advaitists could discover no firm basis for individuality. They compared their finding to the experience of peeling the leaves of a banana tree or an onion. As the layers are pulled off one by one, we are left with only the leaves, piled one around the other. At the end, there is no supporting stem holding it all together. Similarly, our individuality comprises layer upon layer of relative and changeable personality traits, memories, thoughts, and feelings, but there is no absolute reality holding these things together.

Extending their logic further, Advaitists argued that a thing cannot exist if it has only an ill-defined, amorphous reality. There must be something that has concrete reality that lies at the base of things, and from which objects in the world are derived. The base must be unchangeable and indivisible if it is to form the root of all the changes and variety of the world. Using this logic, Advaitists concluded that, behind the fuzzy reality of the world, there is an absolute from which it is derived. Advaitists had similar ideas about individual consciousness. Beyond our fuzzy personal minds, there exists an eternal, unmoving consciousness, of which all these isolated consciousnesses were only a half-formed manifestation.

In this way, Advaita declares that the external world of phenomena and the internal world of consciousness mirror each other. Both have two planes, or layers, of existence; the relative, "unreal" plane and the absolute plane.

Then Advaita makes the vital conclusion, that the absolute that lies at the basis of the external world is the same absolute that lies at the basis of our own consciousness—the Chandogya Upanishad states, "That which is beyond the eye is the same as that which is beyond the sun." The same absolute gives existence and reality to the play of shadows in both the world and in our own consciousness. This absolute, then, is all the reality there is; it is the only thing that exists. Whether we seek truth in the external world or seek it within ourselves, when we strike out all that is temporary and unreal, we will come across the same absolute reality that exists beyond everything. This absolute is Brahman.

> *That great, birthless self is undecaying, immortal, undying, fearless and infinite. Brahman is indeed fearless. He who knows it as such certainly becomes the fearless Brahman.*
> —Brihadaranyaka Upanishad IV.iv.25

In Advaita, this Brahman is the basis of all existence. Everything in the universe is manifested from Brahman and is a limited form of Brahman. The whole universe, all its myriad differences and eternal play, have that one single cause, which is the absolute truth.

The seers of the Upanishads searched for that truth, that principle, which is beyond time and space, beyond cause and effect, eternal and unchanging. Nothing in the universe has these qualities—hence the whole of the universe was rejected as having only relative or partial truth. It is only Brahman, which lies beyond this universe and of which this universe is only a manifestation, that can be of such a nature. Brahman is the absolute truth.

Brahman is one, without parts and absolute; it is not bound by name, form, or causation. The absolute is birthless, changeless, and deathless. It cannot change because it is not a compound. Because there is nothing in the universe different from Brahman, nothing can exert a force that would change it. Birth and death are possible only for that which is compound.

Brahman is not bound by time and space. Time is present only for events, which means change. Space is present only for objects, which are circumscribed. Time and space are intrinsically connected to the manifestation of this universe. But Brahman, which both encompasses and lies beyond the universe, cannot have time and space connected with it.

In addition, Brahman does not have any qualities. Qualities are present for an object—like color, softness, and shape—or for individual consciousness—qualities like misery, and happiness. Brahman does not have any qualities because qualities can be possible only for a circumscribed substance. A color or texture can be present only in an object. Happiness and misery can be present only in an individual consciousness.

Brahman, which is the absolute, cannot have such qualities, as it is not circumscribed in any way and supersedes definition. A quality like redness can be neither present nor absent in Brahman. By virtue of its absoluteness, Brahman rises above these qualities and transcends them. When Brahman is qualified in a certain way, it can manifest as matter with specific properties like redness or softness; however, it can never be adequately described based on these manifestations. Brahman gives rise to different qualities, but cannot be defined by them.

Similarly, Brahman transcends individual consciousness. Individual consciousness can be present only in the relative world because it is present only in relation to others. In our state of consciousness, we must also be aware of the consciousness of others. Because

Brahman is absolute, there is no *other* to be conscious of. But Brahman is not unconscious either; otherwise, consciousness could not have been manifested in the universe. Brahman is unlimited and, hence, is said to have absolute consciousness.

A question may arise as to why we should conceive of a single reality behind this play of variety in the universe. Both the Buddhists and the Advaitists, accept that the world is only a relative reality, but Buddhists go on to say there is no absolute beyond this, and the actual reality is this dance itself, this play of interaction in the universe without anything as the base.

The Advaitist conclusion, that an absolute reality does lie at the base of things, is founded on experiences gathered in meditation. The seers of old experienced a state of merger with the absolute in the deepest state of meditation, *samadhi*, but they also drew on logic to prove its existence. The Mundaka Upanishad says, "By his light all this shines."

If there was not a single base, then this interaction between different objects in the world would not happen. Things can interact with each other only because they have something in common, and it is through this commonality that they react. Two completely different objects would not be able to interact. For example, when two chemicals react, it is because they have the same atomic constituents and energies. If the atoms and energies were of completely different natures they would not relate in any way. There must be something that links cause and effect together.

Again, the Upanishads maintain that things cannot be unreal through and through. Everything we perceive is changing and hence unreal, but Advaita says there must be something real behind this play of unreality. Every object and event in this universe has an ultimate reality behind it. When objects undergo change, they do not do so in a single jump, but in a fluid process, which remains connected to the object throughout the change. Even though the object's state at the end of the process is very different from its state at the beginning, the two states are connected and must have some common bond. For example, if we consider a burning candle, it changes in form to ashes and smoke. Because this change is fluid, there must be something in common between the wax candle, the ashes, and the smoke. In this case, the same atoms and energies from the candle are merely transformed into a different state—ashes, smoke, and radiant energy.

If we are to accept that there is a single basis for all objects in the universe, the single basis, ground, or absolute must remain unchanged. If the ground of being is to remain common, changes must occur only in the nature of the objects that it creates and supports. If the ground itself were to change with each object, then it would not remain a common ground; the base of each object would be different. In that case, there would be no commonality in the universe and the world would be complete chaos. Because the world does have commonalities and is not complete chaos, there must be a single, unchanging absolute that manifests and supports the myriad of differentiated objects we perceive. The Katha Upanishad states, "Through His luster all these are variously illumined." The same effulgent Brahman both creates and forms the basis of this universe; the universe is Brahman itself.

In modern physics, we find that all matter is ultimately constituted of some common subatomic particles, the neutron, proton, and electron. These particles are common to all the manifestations of matter, and it is only their different organization that gives rise to different types of matter. In the example of the candle, it was this material substrate that formed the commonality between the wax, the ashes, and the smoke. The same atoms that were once organized into a candle were organized into ashes and smoke as the candle burned. Even though the universe appears diverse, it has a common source at its base.

Quantum theory has shown that even subatomic particles are composed of smaller, more transitory pieces. It has also shown that matter and energy are basically the same and are interchangeable. Even though matter and energy are, by themselves, two entirely different entities with contradictory properties, they can be transformed into one another, and are therefore part of a spectrum that has some underlying commonality. If they can be changed into each other, then they must have something in common, something of which both are parts. Again, that commonality cannot be just matter or just energy, because both have different properties, but must be something apart and equidistant from both, and from which both can be derived.

When we find that the entire mass-energy present in the universe is part of a spectrum, we are led to the conclusion that there is one source from which it all originates. All the different parts of the spectrum must ultimately be derived from this common base. Because all phenomena themselves are ultimately found to be ill-defined and nebulous, this common base must be something beyond phenomena, and from which all phenomena are only manifestations. Because quantum physics no longer talks about individual particles, but instead about a spectrum of existence, the common base cannot be atomic, but must be a "field" of existence.

This base must remain equidistant from all parts of the spectrum, as all parts are equivalent. It is the changes in the effects that lead to different manifestations, not changes in the cause, which is singular and absolute. The absolute cannot be a part of the universe itself, or it too would be unreal, and hence could not be a common base. To be common to all phenomena, it must remain untouched by any changes in phenomenal existence. A common entity must be changeless. To remain unchanged, it must also exist beyond time and space. This common "base" cannot be bound by time and space, and so it is a common "field," a common ground that is continuous and never divided. The idea that a common basis exists is indicated by the ever-changing nature of reality. The basis must exist *beyond* the universe that emanates from it because the universe is unreal, relative, and ill-defined.

This common base is called Brahman in Advaita. Brahman lies behind and beyond all changes, and, according to the properties it manifests, we experience different forms of existence. The Chandogya Upanishad says: "In the beginning, all this was Existence. One only, without a second." Brahman exists beyond time and space and is the base and the genesis of all that exists in the universe. We have seen that both Advaitic logic and modern science can be used to support the theory that an absolute reality exists beyond our world. . Of course, the Advaitic logic from the Upanishads takes the theory a step further by illustrating that, along with matter and energy, consciousness is derived from Brahman.

Even if we accept that there is a single absolute behind the material world, and also accept that our consciousness is impermanent and there is an absolute behind it, why should we say that the absolute that lies behind the world is the same absolute that lies beyond our own consciousness?

Advaitic philosophers arrived at the conclusion that both absolutes are the same through meditation and logic. Logically, there cannot be two absolute existences. The absolute, by definition, is that which lies beyond all existences; it must be singular. All things in the world, including consciousness, are different but related phenomena. Consciousness is a part of the universe and interacts with it, arising and subsiding within it; it is not an outside phenomenon. Because it is of a different order than insentient or unconscious matter, it is considered to be a different dimension of existence.

But ultimately consciousness is part of the universe, and its root—Brahman—is the same. Consciousness cannot be considered an ephemeral entity without a root cause; it has as much reality as the material world, so it must also have a root cause. Having arisen from the universe, consciousness necessarily has the same cause of origin as the rest of the universe. Because by definition Brahman is the cause of the rest of the universe, it must also be the cause of consciousness. The same absolute lies beyond all phenomena of the universe and gives rise to both material and mental phenomena.

Thus, in the Upanishads, there are two planes or levels of existence—the absolute plane of Brahman and the relative plane of the world, which subsists or sits like a crust on the absolute plane. The relative plane of the world, the crust, exists in three dimensions—material, or *sat*, consciousness, or *chit*, and bliss, or *ananda*. Sat is the material world, including our bodies. Chit is consciousness, both our own and that of all living bodies. Bliss or ananda, which is obtained in meditation, is considered in Hindu psychology to be the true form of consciousness and a higher dimension of existence. These three entities, like three strands interwoven into a cloth, are considered the three dimensions of the relative or superficial plane of existence, the universe. The base of this relative plane of the universe is Brahman. When we remove that which is untrue, we find the existence of Brahman.

One analogy used to describe the relation of Brahman and the world is that of the sea and the wave. All forms of matter and energy and consciousness that exist in the universe are like the waves. The ground of all this existence, Brahman, is like the sea. The waves arise from the sea, but they are not separate from the sea, nor are they composed of anything that is not the sea. The waves are only points in the sea that have acquired a form. That form is recognized in our consciousness where it acquires a name. Once we see the wave, we do not see the sea. But if we can see the wave apart from its name and form, we understand that it was only ever and still is the sea. Moreover, the waves are only temporary; they arise, interact with each other, and again merge into the ground. They have only a relative existence in relation to the sea. The recognition of their existence as a separate entity relies on an observer who sees only name and form, and who cannot distinguish the waves from the sea.

Another useful analogy is that of the snow on the mountain peak. We may initially think that the surface of the snow is the mountain peak, but in reality it is the rock of the mountain underneath that is the real peak. The snow is only a temporary and flimsy covering. Similarly, the green plant layer on the top of a lake might appear to be the surface, but it is the water underneath that is the actual lake. We might think of the sea and icebergs— although they are frozen and look very different, icebergs are still only the sea, and eventually dissolve back into it. We might also think of a sheet of cloth that is creased at some points and flat at others, pots made of earth, whose form does not change their essence, and jewelry made of gold.

The Upanishads are filled with similar comparisons, but it must be realized that these are analogies only and cannot be stretched beyond a certain point; the exact relationship between Brahman and the world in Advaita cannot be described in terms of human experience. In Advaitism, the world manifests from Brahman in the same way as the wave manifests from the sea; however, in Advaita, Brahman produces manifestations that are ill-defined, whereas in the analogies, the waves, pots, and, snow are changed forms of the base, and therefore have a well-defined existence. It is virtually impossible to find an analogy in the world that can give the exact idea of an ill-defined reality. This is because we cannot conceive of anything that has an ill-defined reality. Hence, these analogies are more appropriate for what is known as qualified monism than the non-dualism of Advaita.

Somewhat surprisingly, the best analogy describing the relationship between the world and Brahman comes from quantum physics. Here, too, the fundamental constituents of the universe, subatomic particles, do not have a true reality but are only hazy entities. An electron, for example, does not exist as a true particle, but only as a cloud of possibility. Other particles and forces have the same kind of fuzzy reality. Quantum physicists are emphatic that the reality of the world they describe cannot be understood by the human mind; it is a nebulous existence beyond our conception. This "ill-defined reality" of the world is precisely what Advaita seeks to explain.

The reality of the world is subject to change and is of a nebulous nature, whereas the reality of Brahman is absolute. In considering the mass of a body, for example, we can easily see that it is relative. We cannot assign a figure for the mass that will prove true in all circumstances. Whenever we describe the mass of a body, we have to define it in terms of our measurement. The mass may have been measured at rest, or in one particular coordinate.

Depending on tools and conditions, the same object will produce different measurements of mass, yet none of these different masses are truer; they are all equally true. Thus no object has an absolute mass true for all aspects. Similarly, no object has an absolute length, breadth, or speed.

This relativism holds true for the laws of physics as well. No laws are absolutely true. Isaac Newton's laws of motion were considered absolute truth, but we now know that they are true only when they are applied to objects moving more slowly than the speed of light. If an object's speed is greater, we have to consider the relativistic laws of motion. Similarly, it is very likely that the relativistic laws are only true under certain conditions and are not absolutely true, as, for example, when we consider the effects of gravity.

However, in contemporary physics, there are some values that are considered to be absolutely true—such as the speed of light, which is considered constant in all circumstances. Though the speed of light is considered unchanging for all purposes today, no one would seriously guarantee that it is really an absolute truth. Further progress of science may well show us that this too, is only relative.

In the Advaitic view, all that exists in this universe has relative truth only, and is a manifestation of the absolute truth, Brahman. This concept of relative and absolute truth becomes vital when we consider it in the sphere of consciousness. It means that our individual consciousness also has only a relative reality and its basis is the absolute Brahman. Hence, our true identity is not our individual consciousness but Brahman, and we can realize this in a mystical experience by subsuming our individual identity in the absolute.

He who inhabits the earth, but is within it, whom the earth does not know, whose body is the earth, and who controls the earth from within, is the internal ruler, your own immortal self.

—Brihadaranyaka Upanishad III.vii.2

What does the term absolute mean in relation to Brahman? How do we conceive of the absolute? We call Brahman absolute because it is beyond all changes, all relativity, all qualities, and all differentiation, but the precise nature of absolute existence is something we cannot understand. By virtue of human development, our minds are trained to understand this world. We function in the presence of this world, and our consciousness has developed to make sense of this world only. We are only able to understand relative reality, relative space, and relative time. We must make comparisons between differentiated forms to understand them, and can therefore only possess relative knowledge. We cannot understand absolute knowledge not bound by *upadhis*, or limitations. We cannot grasp a concept beyond time and space, beyond all qualities and change. Nor can we find words to describe Brahman. The language we use is dependent on the concepts we have in our minds and is bound up with the relative world. There is no way to describe the absolute. Brahman is "that from which all words turn back."

In one meditation, the mantra used to describe the Absolute is the famous "neti, neti," or, "not this, not this," of the Brhadaranyaka Upanishad. Here, the main idea is that Brahman is both indescribable and inconceivable. No concept we have or might develop will ever be sufficient to describe Brahman, so it is best to negate all concepts that may arise by saying, "not this, not this." The absolute is ineffable, beyond human conception.

Because the mind can never form an accurate conception of the absolute, we can only become one with Brahman by becoming free of our minds. The Upanishad tells us to leave behind all religion, all scriptures, leave behind even the Upanishads to achieve Brahman. Only when we achieve a state that rises higher than all our worldly conceptions can we achieve knowledge or oneness with Brahman.

It is important to understand that this concept of the absolute is not valueless just because we are not able to conceive of it in terms of human thoughts. In physics, too, we encounter several concepts not readily encompassed by the human imagination, but physicists manage to deal with them every day. A concept cannot be dismissed as meaningless or worthless simply because it is not easily imagined by the human mind. In Advaita, we *can* achieve knowledge of Brahman, but in a state higher than our ordinary worldly consciousness.

We might also ask how Brahman gives origin to the world. If Brahman is the cause and the world is the effect, how is the world generated from Brahman?

Because Brahman cannot be encompassed by our words, the answer can only be given by analogies. No analogy can be perfect, for no analogy can touch Brahman; however, the Upanishad's description of interactions between light and jewels is useful for understanding how the world emanates from Brahman. When white light is shone on a red jewel, it transmits only red light. The white light itself is not changed; a part of the light is transmitted, and this limited part appears red. The red light cannot be called a changed form of the white light, because it is only a small piece of the white light. When the white light is limited, it gives rise to the red. Here, Brahman is the white light and the world the red light. Brahman is not changed into the world, but is differentiated and limited in the process of making the world manifest. Brahman gives rise to the world, but never changes into it.

What plays the role of the jewel in this analogy? The Upanishads define them as upadhis. Upadhis are the qualifiers and limitations that enable the manifestation of the world. When Brahman is qualified by one upadhi, it gives rise to a rock. When qualified by another, it may give rise to air. Yet another upadhi will give rise to the human body and its consciousness. The boundaries set by upadhis give us the different objects in the universe and all their different qualities.

Of course, like analogies used to describe Brahman's relationship to the world, analogies used to describe how the world emanates from Brahman do not provide an accurate picture of Advaitic theory, and work better for qualified monism. In Advaita, Brahman's transformations into worldly phenomena are only apparent changes. The world is ill-defined and fuzzy, unlike the examples in analogies. No analogy can truly describe how Brahman is changed into the world, because all analogies must express relationships between objects in this world. They can never express relationships to something beyond the whole existence.

All objects and properties that exist in the relative universe arise from the differentiation of Brahman. There is nothing in the universe that is not Brahman, although in a limited state. The universe is complex and ever-changing. It is subject to death, birth, and decay. Because nothing in the universe is absolute, there can be no absolute knowledge of any part. But if we can know Brahman, we can know that which is the basis. If we can achieve knowledge of Brahman, we no longer need to know each individual facet of the universe, for we will arrive at the root. By knowing Brahman, we can know everything in this world.

What exactly is meant when we say the world has only relative (or fuzzy) existence? What is the nature of this relative existence? Advaitic philosophy explains that the world is relative and ill-defined because it has properties of both existence and nonexistence. The world has properties of existence because it does exist, at least relatively, but it also has properties of nonexistence because it has no absolute reality. When Advaita asserts that the world is unreal, this does not mean that it doesn't exist, but that it does not have any absolutes. This universal law—that the world exists but has no absolute reality—is called *maya*, and maya is inexplicable. We can never fully conceptualize the nature of this half-real world, but we know that maya is its nature.

Maya, the nature of the world, is often defined as illusion. It is like a mirage; we cannot deny that a mirage exists, yet it has no reality in itself. It is also like a dream. As long as we are inside it, the world seems real, but once we are removed, incongruities are apparent, and a formerly logical, constructed world becomes nothing but a mass of confusion. Buddhists compare the concept of maya to the circle of fire produced by a whirling firebrand. Though a quickly turning firebrand appears to create a fiery ring in the air, the circle is really only an illusion created by movement.

All these analogies are common to both Advaitism and Buddhism, both of which regard the world as having only a relative reality. The difference is that in Buddhism, the world is said to be unreal through and through; there is no absolute behind it, and maya is a true illusion. In Advaitism, the phenomenal world is maya, but the reality of Brahman lies beyond it. The Advaitist recognizes that even the mirage needs an oasis, the dream, a waking world, and the circle of fire, a firebrand. In the same way, the relative world needs Brahman. Just as we experience a whirling firebrand as a circle of fire, we experience Brahman as the world. In Advaitism, the concept of maya does not mean illusion alone, but takes into account both relative and absolute modes of existence.

Modern physics also has difficulty explaining the nature of relative existence. Time and space are ultimately dependent on an observer, yet we cannot say that time and space do not exist. Because time and space are relative, their exact natures cannot be known; we can only say they exist conditionally. Similarly, it is difficult for physics to satisfactorily define the natures of matter and energy. Subatomic entities are contradictory, existing as both particle and wave. Science must finally adopt a worldview that includes an understanding of existence very similar to the Advaitist and Buddhist concept of maya.

In another, broader, sense, maya also signifies, not just that the world is an illusion, but the entrancing quality of this illusion, which has trapped us all so firmly that it is almost impossible to get out of its clutches. The dual existence of good and bad, our constant search for an elusive happiness, love of wealth, our desperate clutching to the lives of ourselves and our kin even when we know that it will surely end—all this is maya. As long as we are in her grip, we will never see beyond illusion. Religion is but an attempt to cut free.

An important question that arises is, if we are Brahman, why do we not know it already? Why should we believe that we are our individual identities? Advaita teaches that maya's powers of delusion prevent us from recognizing our true nature as Brahman. Maya, the entrancing illusion of the world, ensures that we understand individual consciousness and the external world as true entities instead of recognizing them as merely relative. This delusion arises at birth and is consolidated by our experiences thereafter. A new-born baby does not come into the world with a clean slate, but carries evolutionary impressions and instincts that will allow it to survive as a human in this world. As the baby grows older, it begins the process of learning and acquires its sense of ego. All its knowledge and consciousness are irretrievably tied to the perspective of this ego. All humans live and learn within the small sphere of experience compatible with our senses and understanding. All understanding of the world is completely bound to individual perception.

The delusion that maya inspires is called *avidya*, meaning "ignorance" or "without knowledge" in Sanskrit. If we can break away from avidya we will discover our true identity and the delusion will fall away. The Upanishads make this claim over and over again. Though we appear to be trapped in individual consciousness, we can break the chain of delusion and realize that we are the absolute, Brahman. Our personalities are bound up in thousands of fears, desires, and hopes. We find ourselves entangled in all these only because we identify with our personalities rather than with our true nature. If we recognize that we are, in fact, the absolute, then fears and desires count for nothing.

The Hindu sage and mystic Ramakrishna Paramahamsa (1836–1886) used the story of a lion raised by sheep to illustrate avidya. While the lion lived among the sheep, he considered himself a sheep and behaved like one, eating grass and roaming. One day, a passing lion saw him and told him that he was actually a lion. He ran to the river, looked at his reflection, and realized that he was indeed a lion and not a sheep. He looked up and, for the first time in his life, roared out. Thereafter, he never again behaved like a sheep, but acted like the lion that he was. Like the lion, once we realize our true nature, we will no longer be content with our individual identity—we will have the strength of Brahman.

This Self is the ruler of all beings, and the king of all beings. Just as all the spokes are fixed on the nave and the felloe of a chariot wheel, so are all the beings, all gods, all worlds, all organs and all these individual selves fixed in this Self.

—Brihadaranyaka Upanishad II.iv.14

The nature of Brahman's transformation into the world is a fundamental point in Advaita. For Advaitists, this change is *vivartavada*, or unreal, and only an apparent modification. It is not the real modification, or *parinamavada*, of the qualified monists. The belief that Brahman's transformation is only an apparent one clearly distinguishes the true monism of Advaita from philosophies of qualified monism. Advaita maintains that the change is unreal because the world itself is an illusion.

Because the world has no absolute reality, Brahman's change into the world is true only on a relative scale. Name and form change, but these changes only hold true in a system of subject-object duality. Because Brahman's essence remains unchanged, on the absolute scale the world is still Brahman. We will see the world only as long as we are bound by our relative viewpoint; thus, on the absolute scale, the change is unreal or apparent (i.e., vivartavada). This is important especially for individual consciousness, because it means that we do not change into our personalities, but remain Brahman; hence we can regain the identity of Brahman.

If the world does have existence, even if only relative, then why do we say that Brahman is part-less or quality-less? If we say that the world has evolved from Brahman, then it would mean that the world is a part or an effect of Brahman, but the effect is always the cause in a changed form. In this case, Brahman cannot be considered changeless. As all qualities of the world are part of Brahman, Brahman cannot be considered quality-less either. Because Brahman changes into the world, it should be affected by time and space. The world's presence seems to contradict the absoluteness of Brahman.

In fact, the two are not contradictory, due to the unreality of the world, as it is understood in Advaita. Because the world has only relative reality, it is untrue on the absolute scale. Brahman is absolute even though it has an effect—the world—*because the effect is not truly real*. With this vital illumination, Advaita defines Brahman as absolute, unchanged, and so forth, even though it has the world as an effect. There is no change in Brahman; the change is only apparent, or vivartavada. Even though the world is affected by time, space, and causation, these qualities apply in the world only on the relative scale. On the absolute scale, the world itself is false, and so Brahman is not affected.

It is important to understand that Advaita does not claim that the world is totally unreal or that it does not exist; it only says that the world has a lower grade of reality. Advaita maintains that the world and Brahman have two grades of reality. Brahman is true from all aspects (that is, it has absolute reality), while the world is true only in relation to an observer. Even during un-manifested epochs, the world continues to exist in a seed form, as a potential only, in Brahman. This understanding of Brahman's absolute reality is why Advaita is defined as non-dual philosophy, and not monism. In Advaita both the world and Brahman are recognized, but because the world does not have a true existence, Brahman alone is true; hence there is non-duality. Once the merely relative reality of this world has been logically proven, the rest of Advaitic philosophy, both metaphysical theory and practice, follows naturally.

Another question that might arise is, why does Brahman evolve into the world? Since Brahman is absolute and unchanged by the world, and therefore the question does not arise of Brahman willing or creating the universe, then what causes the evolution of the world?

The answer is a vital part of Advaitic theory: the universe passes through the cosmic cycle, the cycle of Brahman. According to traditional Indian thought, this cycle is considered to be a single "day of Brahma." The day of Brahma is a period of time when the universe is seen in its relative existence as a manifested presence. The night of Brahma is the time when the universe remains involute, or in the un-manifested state.

This cosmic cycle is not a willed process, but a natural circuit through which the universe passes. Brahman does not set the cycle in motion; it is simply part of the nature of the universe. This makes Advaita the most naturalistic theory of religious metaphysics; there is nothing to direct this cycle or to control it. The universe has been passing through this cycle forever, and it will continue to pass through it for all the years to come. Advaita does not address why the universe moves in cycles, but considers them very important because they enable relative existence. The cycle of expansion and manifestation is called *pravritti*. It is like a growing circle, or a dilating ripple in a pond. The reverse movement of the cycle is called *nivritti*. The circle shrinks, becoming progressively smaller, until it eventually becomes un-manifest.

It is important to note that this cycle does not affect Brahman, but affects the relative universe. Brahman never undergoes the changes this cycle brings, because change and its effects are unreal. Because we live on the relative plane, we experience change, but if we were able to break from our relative viewpoint and see things on the absolute scale, change would disappear. On the scale of Brahman, change does not occur.

During the time of involution, the world remains in an unmanifested state, as a seed in Brahman. The world doesn't become nonexistent at the time of involution, as it would fail to be manifested again, but the upadhis, or limiting adjuncts, remain in potential form and are not expressed. As expansion begins again, the upadhis are expressed and cause the manifestation of the relative universe. In this way, the cycle goes on.

An infinite number of cycles of Brahman have occurred. There is no beginning or end to this cycle as long as we are caught up in the relative world. Only if we break out of relativity and become one with the absolute will we be able to realize the illusory nature of this cycle.

Again, we may ask, what is the point of all the arguments about whether the world is real or only apparently real? Advaitists have spent a great deal of energy showing that the world is ill-defined, relative, and not a true reality. A qualified monist might ask, what is the harm in saying that Brahman's transformation into the universe is a real change instead of an apparent change? Isn't the difference only in the choice of words used?

Although the difference between real and apparent change may seem, at first, like verbal quibbling, this is not so at all, as everything changes with this definition. The entire philosophy of Advaita stands on the tenet that change and its effects are unreal.

In qualified monism, Brahman's change into the world is real, and so the world is real. This is a completely different metaphysical viewpoint. Advaita reasons that if Brahman is the absolute, then the world, which is based on it, can have only a relative reality, and this view is logically consistent. Modern science agrees, accepting the relative nature of the world rather than the static reality of old Newtonian physics. The Advaitic view of vivartavada—the assertion that change is only apparent—is both more logical and more in agreement with contemporary science. The evidence contradicts the theory of parinamavada, that the nature of the world is real; so, from a purely philosophical viewpoint, Advaita metaphysics is superior to other positions.

For practical religious practice, the idea that change is real means that there is a higher and lower existence in qualified monism. If Brahman is truly changed when the world manifests, Brahman and the world are dual entities with separate and equally real realities. The world becomes a lower form of Brahman, a part, and Brahman remains the higher form, the whole. This leads to the concept of a personal god who controls us and to whom we can pray.

In Advaita, because change is not real, there is no god higher than us; we ourselves are the absolute and control our own destiny. The goals of mystical experience in dualism, qualified monism, and Advaita are different because of varying beliefs regarding the reality of the phenomenal, changing world. Dualists see visions of God or hear God speaking. Qualified monists experience God's contact or feel God suffusing them without losing personal identity. They are always separate from the absolute. But in Advaita, the aspirant *is* the absolute. The Advaitists go a step further, completely losing individualism and regaining identity as the absolute. The goal of Advaita is thus the ultimate mystical experience.

When seen through the lens of Advaita, the universe itself becomes holy; the sun, the moon, and the stars—everything is holy because everything has Brahman at its base. Every man, woman, and child is holy, because we all have Brahman as our base. Everything around us becomes an object for our veneration. This is what takes Advaita further than pure science and makes it a spiritual quest.

The concept that the same absolute lies behind everything in the universe, including us, forms the basis of Advaitic logic, metaphysics, ethics, and practice. It is also the basis of Advaitic mysticism—if we can break out of relativity, we can experience our true, absolute self. Advaitic ethics is derived from the conception that everything is one. A person who has this knowledge would only do that which benefits all. This forms the basic ethical principle that what is selfish is evil and what is unselfish is good. Again, Advaita provides the basis for answers such as who we are, where we have come from, and where we are heading. It gives us a goal, which is to know our true identity, Brahman.

> *This self of mine within the heart, is smaller than a paddy or barley or mustard or a syamaka seed. This self of mine within the heart, is greater than this earth, greater than the intermediate space, greater than heaven, greater than all these worlds.*
> —Chandogya Upanishad III.xiv.3

Consciousness is undoubtedly one of the biggest quandaries that faces us when we try to understand the world. Our consciousness is what really defines us. Our bodies, our social relations, even our actions, do not satisfactorily define us. What defines us is our "I-ness," our sense of self, and the impressions, thoughts, and sensations that we have. When we talk of knowing ourselves, it is our consciousness that we seek to know.

Consciousness is of a different order of existence than material existence. This fact confronts us immediately when we consider it. A conscious entity has awareness; it is aware of itself and aware of the external elements. A nonconscious body is not similarly aware. We may argue regarding the nature of this awareness, but we certainly cannot say that it does not exist. We must grant a difference between a conscious and a nonconscious body.

The most common way of understanding consciousness among religions is the concept of the soul, which is the seat of individual consciousness. The soul is a nonmaterial entity, which is present in the body and is the conscious part of our existence. It receives sensations from the body and in turn directs the body to move and perform other actions.

Different religions understand the soul in different ways. In dualism, the soul exists as a real entity, completely different from God in both substance and form. In qualified monism, the soul is a real entity and the seat of consciousness, but it has a divine nature. The soul is said to be a spark from God.

Defining each individual consciousness as a separate entity leads to questions about how consciousness interacts with the body, how it evolved, and at which level of animal life it exists. But individual consciousness is understood differently in Advaita. In Advaita, individual consciousness is not separate from the material universe. Both exist on the same plane. As with the material world, when individual consciousness exists on the relative plane, it is unreal, but it is recognizable as our individual identity. Behind this is the absolute, Brahman.

Qualified in one way, Brahman gives rise to material existence; qualified another, it gives rise to individual consciousness. Just as Brahman supports the universe's material existence on the material plane, Brahman supports all personal thoughts and sensations on the plane of consciousness. Individual consciousness, the body, and the brain are all produced by the upadhis and manifestations of Brahman. Our individual consciousness, like everything in the universe, exists only in this realm of maya. Consciousness and matter (and bliss, the third strand) are like strands of a rope or cloth interwoven together in the universe, at the base of both of which is the absolute of Brahman.

This understanding of individual consciousness is based on the meditative findings of sages. They declared that consciousness is nothing but a complex of "I-ness"-thought-sensations. When we analyze our minds, we cannot find any "I-ness" apart from our thoughts and sensations. When we analyze our thoughts and sensations, we always find that a sense of "I-ness" is an integral part of them.

When we can control our thoughts and awareness, individual consciousness disintegrates. But the result is not a blank, because at the basis of individual consciousness is Brahman. When we can control our individual consciousness and make it fade away, the consciousness of Brahman manifests itself. We then realize that what we took for our individual consciousness was a shadow only, a false existence; the true existence is this absolute consciousness.

Thus, even if we define the soul, or *atman*, as the seat of our individual consciousness, this atman in Advaita is not a separate real existence but a relative existence only. Atman here is only a name for individual consciousness. The atman, individual consciousness or the ego-thoughts-sensations complex exists only on the relative plane and has no absolute truth. Because it does not define the soul or consciousness as true entities, Advaita is the most scientific of all religious theories regarding consciousness. Advaitists can easily accept that the brain supports consciousness, because the body and individual consciousness coexist on the same relative and limited plane. But, of course, the *base* of consciousness in Advaita is not the brain but Brahman.

Brahman is not affected by the changes in our consciousness. The changes in our everyday lives occur only at the level of our own consciousness. Because Brahman is the basis of all consciousness, it is not affected by the individual changes. All events in our minds—the emotions of anger and happiness, our selfish or selfless intentions—are all on the plane of maya and do not have any true reality. They cannot affect Brahman, the root of all that is in the universe.

Because consciousness is produced from Brahman, it means that Brahman cannot be devoid of consciousness. It signifies that Brahman has the potentiality of consciousness; that is, it can be qualified in a certain way so that it produces consciousness. Though Brahman can produce consciousness, it does not have an individual consciousness because individual consciousness can only be perceived from a limited viewpoint. Instead, Brahman has absolute consciousness, which is higher than and contains individual consciousness.

In the Upanishads, three qualities are ascribed to Brahman. Brahman is existence, consciousness, and bliss, or "*Satchitananda.*" Nothing can exist which is not a manifestation from Brahman and whose properties are not already present in Brahman. Existence, consciousness, and bliss are the three cardinal properties of the universe and the three modes in which Brahman manifests in the universe. Existence, or *sat*, is the quality of all material things, and Brahman lies as the basis of this existence. Individual consciousness, or *cit*, is another fundamental quality of the universe, experienced as personal identity. In Hindu psychology, bliss, or *ananda*, is the cardinal property and purest state of individual consciousness, and it is given a separate status as important as consciousness.

All other emotions and thoughts, like anger, sadness, or grief, are degradations of pure bliss and do not have independent existence. When the mind moves outward, we experience other emotions and feelings, but when the mind is pure, we experience true bliss. Existence, consciousness, and bliss define the universe and are present in Brahman, but even these three cardinal properties of the universe are ultimately limited and relative. They are constantly changing and impermanent. Because they are derived from the absolute Brahman, Brahman is said to have absolute existence, absolute consciousness, and absolute bliss.

But again, this does not mean that the absolute can be defined by three qualities. When we study Brahman, as we must, from the standpoint of individual consciousness, we ascribe a quality like absolute consciousness to it. We use this terminology, but, of course, consciousness is possible only on the relative scale; there cannot be anything like absolute consciousness—it is simply a word that we use to describe the transcendence of Brahman. This is similarly the case for the terms absolute existence and absolute bliss.

Qualities such as absolute bliss, absolute existence, and absolute consciousness are ascribed to Brahman only for the purposes of meditation and reasoning. When we consider Brahman, we must always do so from the standpoint of our own selves, so we see Brahman as having the qualities that define us. In the initial stages of meditation, we see Brahman from our relative standpoint, and hence Brahman appears as having these three cardinal qualities. It is only in the final *samadhi*, *Nirvikalpa Samadhi*, when we break out totally from the relative viewpoint, that we will see Brahman as free from all qualities.

The Advaitic conception of Brahman is the final conception of metaphysics, the ultimate reductionist philosophy. The Prasna Upanishad says: "This is all. Beyond this there is nothing." Brahman, by definition, is the ultimate generalization. There cannot be any further reduction than the absolute Brahman, which is conceived of as a singularity. Advaita is therefore also the simplest and the purest of all philosophies. There is no particular article of faith on which Advaitism depends for survival. Advaitists can declare their independence from all books, teachers, and religions, because, ultimately, they do not depend on any dogmatic position for their teachings. Advaita is the most powerful of all conceptions of truth.

As defined by Advaita, the absolute is something that could be easily accepted by scientists. The position that there is an absolute from which all this universe is manifested, and that is itself beyond all changes, does not contradict scientific thought, and quantum mechanics appears to be heading in the direction of just such a view. The Advaitic explanation of the origin of the universe—that it moves in unwilled, natural cycles of manifestation and un-manifestation—is remarkably similar to contemporary scientific views. Most scientists accepting such a view would still consider themselves atheists, yet Advaita is a religious path and not just a simple scientific view of the universe.

This is because Advaita defines Brahman as the basis for the existence not just of the external world, but of the internal world also—as the basis for our own existence. Because Brahman has the potentiality of consciousness, it is not an unconscious principle. Rather, Brahman supersedes consciousness and can be described as having unlimited consciousness. Modern science would accept a principle like Brahman as the basis for existence of the external world, but might not consider it for the internal world.

Brahman, which is the ground of all the phenomena that we perceive, is also the ground of our own selves. It is the ground of both the external and the internal. There is therefore no ultimate difference between the external and the internal, no difference between subject and object—there is no duality at all. The Upanishads finally unite everything, including our innermost selves and the outer world, into one. In reality, we ourselves are Brahman; it is only because of our limited capacities that we do not realize this truth. Hence Advaitism also provides an explanation for the basis of mystical experience. Mystical experiences occur when we can be one with the absolute, an experience that is not in the domain of science.

With all this understanding of the world, one question that must be considered, which is most important to us individually, is what happens to us during and after death. Is death really a permanent end to us and all our memories and experiences?

No one, neither an Advaitist, a Christian, nor a Muslim, has ever come back from death. No matter what our beliefs and practices, we will never come back from the dead either. This finality is the one fact about death about which we can be sure. Without any knowledge from the other side, all speculations about death, whether from Advaita or any other religion, must necessarily be speculation only.

The beliefs of dualistic and qualified monism are not entirely satisfactory to our reason. The concept of souls is difficult enough to understand in a living body; the extravagant accounts of what they go through on death are even more difficult to accept. They seem to depend on little other than imagination for their basis, without any firm logic or arguments in their support. These are simple-minded doctrines created purely to appeal to our belief systems.

I am the endless cosmic serpent,
The Lord of all sea creatures,
I am chief of the ancestral fathers;
Among restraints, I am death.

—Bhagavad Gita 10.29

The final explanation given for death is that of monism, that of the Advaita. Advaita explains death on the basis of its metaphysical theories and the beliefs on the relation of God and humans. In Advaita, death is not a contraction but an expansion, an expansion of our individual identity into the Brahman. In death, we finally become one with Brahman.

The Chandogya Upanishad describes death: "O good looking one, of this person when he dies, the organ of speech is withdrawn into the mind, mind into the vital force, vital force into the fire and fire into the Supreme Deity."

The supreme deity here is Brahman. This passage means that as a person dies, his or her mind slowly fades out, thus leaving the true identity more and more pure, until finally, when the differentiation of the mind has ceased completely, the individual consciousness disappears completely and the absolute consciousness of Brahman emerges. "Then, this one who is fully serene, rising up from this body and reaching the highest light, remains established in his true nature. This is the Self. This is Immortal. This is Brahman. Truth is the name of this Brahman who is such."

The individual person reaches "the highest light,"—that is, the light of Brahman—and remains "established in his true nature," that is, Brahman. Thus the person, when he or she dies, attains the nature of Brahman, which is his or her true nature.

Commentators on the Upanishads usually interpret these Upanishadic passages as being true only for the person of knowledge; for the person of ignorance this merger is not complete, and he or she returns from the merger to take up residence in another body, as a reincarnation. A strict interpretation of the Upanishads from an Advaitic viewpoint cannot support this. Good or evil, knowledge or ignorance, is a part of the human mind. When the mind ceases and its differentiation of the absolute consciousness ceases, these notions of knowledge and ignorance die out with it. That which was the differentiation in our personality dies out, and that which was the truth, the absolute Brahman, remains.

The analogy given here in the Chandogya Upanishad is the merger of the nectar of different flowers into honey. "As bees make honey by collecting the essences of different trees standing in different quarters, and reduce the juice into a homogenous whole ... and as they do not have such distinctive ideas as, 'I am the juice of this tree,' 'I am the juice of that tree,' so also, O good looking one, all these creatures, after merging into existence, do not understand this."

Once it is merged into honey, the individual differentiation ceases. Another analogy given is that of the merger of rivers into the sea: "As they do not realize there, 'I am this river,' 'I am that river,' in this very way indeed."

The idea is repeated throughout the scriptures. The Brihadaranyaka Upanishad says, "Being but Brahman, he is merged into Brahman." "Just as the lifeless slough of a snake lies in the anthill, so does this body lie. Then the Self becomes disembodied and immortal, becomes the Prana, becomes the Brahman." The Brahma sutras say, "(When the Jiva) has attained (the highest light) there is manifestation (of its real nature)" and "(The Jiva in the state of liberation exists) as inseparable (from Brahman)."

The main point to consider here is what we think our identity to be. If we think ourselves to be the individual identity, then death is certain for us, as our individuality cannot survive without the mind or the brain. Our individuality is no doubt formed in the brain itself, in its memories and workings, and it cannot survive its disintegration.

But in Advaita, our real nature is not our individual identity but the absolute Brahman. This absolute, limited by the upadhis, gives rise to the individual consciousness. It is Brahman itself, which is manifested as our individual consciousness. Hence the root of our consciousness is the Brahman. As the body dies, the brain will also begin to die. Then the differentiation of the brain will gradually fade away. As all differentiation of the brain ceases, all limitation will cease and our self, our "identity," will expand as it is freed until it becomes one with Brahman. Death then in Advaita is not a contraction of the consciousness but an expansion, the final, long-awaited freedom that we thirst for.

Thus the death of our individual consciousness does not lead into blankness. It leads to the consciousness of Brahman. What exactly this means cannot be described in words, but a parallel can be found in the accounts of mystical experiences of Advaita, where basically the same process is gone through by an active effort during life. Here there is no void when the ego disappears, but instead an unlimited freedom and bliss, which is said to be indescribable. The process of our knowing and understanding is limited to our relative world; we cannot conceive of the absolute consciousness. Our death will also be total in the sense that our relative individuality will fade out. We will certainly not be able to come back, as our "I" will have died out with the brain and mind of the body. But our "I-ness" itself was a falsity, a dead weight to our freedom.

Instead we will regain the freedom of our real nature, from which we were kept away by our delusion and false belief.

The concept of individual consciousness or soul having only temporary reality gives us the fundamental purpose of Advaita, which is to realize the true nature of our selves. In Advaita, what we consider to be our individual identity is merely a relative manifestation from Brahman. Our true identity is Brahman itself. We are never different from Brahman, the difference is only apparent. If we can break out of this shell of relativity, we would find that we are in fact Brahman.

"*Tat tvam asi*—Thou art *That*," says the famous sutra of the Chandogya Upanishad. The Brihadaranyaka Upanishad says, "*Aham Brahmasvi*—I am Brahman."

The absolute toward which all metaphysical speculation is directed, that which is beyond all this illusion, is not outside us but within us. We are already that absolute. Brahman is not something that we need to search for, but rather it is our own selves. It is our true identity. Here in Advaita is the highest point of all philosophy: that the absolute, which lies at the basis of all the external world, is also the basis of our internal world. There is no external or internal world; there is only one truth, and I myself am that absolute truth.

You are the absolute, says the Advaitist. You are God. There is none for you to depend on, none who can help you, and none who can control you. You are your own destiny. You are immutable, eternal, and immortal. You are not bound by time and space, nor are you affected by causation. What then should one who is indestructible be afraid of? Who can harm you, or restrict you? For those who know their true identity, there can be no fear, desire, or sorrow.

Advaita is the most powerful of all philosophies. It promises an ideal of supreme strength to each individual. For the Advaitists, there is no God to turn to, none to guide them, and none who can punish or reward them. Each of us have already this force within us, and need no other's help in our search for the truth. The Advaita also gives the greatest freedom to the individual. For the absolute, there can be no restriction or bondage. All of our efforts are bound in searching for this true freedom, so that there will be nothing that can ever restrict us. But Advaita says this freedom is already ours; we need to only recognize that we have it.

This is the highest position that can be taken for the human soul, and one that is beyond all religions. What religion can there be for one who is the absolute? The Advaita is a revolutionary philosophy, as it negates all other philosophies including itself. The truth is not to be found in logic and arguments, or even by knowing the Vedas or the Upanishads. The truth is already within each of us, and it is only for us to find our true identity.

Religions and their practices are necessary in Advaita, but only as peripheral aids and for the final truth, they must be left behind. The search for the truth in Advaita is a lone search, in which the aspirant has to contend with his or her own self and the delusion associated with it. Such a position weakens organized religions and their doctrines, and hence was regarded with fear and distrust. Advaita was considered to be a secret philosophy in India, meant only for the few who would be able to withstand its shattering ideas. And the thrust of Advaita has always been that, to shatter our comfort in living within this world and lead us to search for our true identity.

This is the final message of Advaita. It is a system of knowledge that seeks to establish the truth behind this world. There are many in the world from time immemorial that have sought only for this truth and nothing else. For them the world has no value. The path shown by the Yogis is a lonely path, meant only for the few among us who have this unquenched desire for the truth and are ready to leave behind everything for this search. The Brihada-ranyaka Upanishad says, "the Self should be realized—should be heard of, reflected on and meditated upon." The Advaita speaks of this self only and of this goal. Its message resounds wherever this search for the truth is embarked upon.

Advaita Compared
to Other Philosophies

*The Self which has no sin, no decrepitude, no death, no sorrow,
no hunger, no thirst, has unfailing desires, unfailing will—
that has to be known. That has to be enquired into. He who,
after knowing the self realizes it, attains all the world and all
the desires.*

—Chandogya Upanishad VIII.vii.1

The Vedas are the source of Hindu religion. They comprise a huge volume of literature and an innumerable number of doctrines can be derived from them. Six schools of philosophy ultimately came to be recognized as the main schools of Hindu philosophy. They are grouped into pairs: *Nyaya* and *Vaisesika*, *Samkhya* and Yoga, and the *Purva Mimamsa* and *Vedanta*. Of these, however, the Vedantic school gained the most prominence; today, Vedic philosophy in general means the Vedantic philosophy. Vedanta again comprises three main divisions: the dualistic, qualified monoistic, and the monistic or advaitic. Upanishadic philosophy is hence not synonymous with Advaitic philosophy; Advaitism is only one of the three offshoots from the Upanishads.

Aside from these six schools based on the Vedas, two other important religions developed in India, Buddhism and Jainism. These schools are not based on the Vedas and hence are not considered part of Hinduism, but in essence most Hindus regard Buddha as one more saint of the Hindu pantheon and regard his teachings as sacred. Jainism too has always been very close to Hinduism, and Jain temples have traditionally been visited by Hindus and vice versa without any hesitation.

To understand Indian thought, it is necessary to have an overview of all these systems.

Nyaya and Vaisesika Schools

The Nyaya and Vaisesika schools are usually studied together. The importance of these two schools lies in that they both took the questions of philosophy and tried to solve them with rational and logical examination. The phenomena of the world were analyzed, and a theory regarding the true metaphysical explanation of the world was derived from this analysis. These schools studied the knowledge that we have of this world and whether we can derive a consistent explanation of the world based on this knowledge. The Nyaya takes as its subject the knowledge within—that is, knowledge gained by analysis and thought—whereas the Vaisesika takes up the knowledge without—that is, knowledge gained through experience. The schools otherwise have common belief systems and both agree on most subjects.

Nyaya became essentially a school of logic, and logic was its most important sphere of study. The study of logic depended on the study of dialectics, or the methods used in arguments. From this study, the Nyayikas developed a system of knowledge, which clarified greatly the way in which we organize what we know.

Nyaya philosophy is essentially based on epistemology, the

philosophy of knowledge. Nyaya began by an impartial inquiry into the contents of our knowledge, rather than the objects; that is, it studied the internal part of our knowledge rather than the external world that inspires it. In doing so, the Nyayikas critically examined the statements regarding our knowledge and subjected them to logical analysis. The Nyayikas were able to create a systemic classification of knowledge and expose intricate details of fallacies and so forth.. The strength of this logical system strengthened the whole of Hindu logic, which always relied on its positions and terms, and all Hindu philosophy was argued on the basis of this logic.

The intricacies of latter Nyaya study are well known, and even among hardened Sanskrit scholars, used as they are to the finest hair-splitting, the Nyaya texts are an object of wonder and fear. However it is a moot question whether the Nyayikas have any role to play beyond the study of logic and epistemology.

If Nyaya logic was strong, Nyaya metaphysics was its weakness. The Nyaya philosophy is a dualist one in which a sharp distinction is made between matter and spirit and between mind and body, and these two dualities are believed to make up the universe.

The Nyayas accepted uncritically the Vaisesika theory of atoms as the basis of the natural world. The world in this theory consists of an innumerable quantity of atoms that are eternal and unchanging, and which in various combinations create this world of nature. The real subject of our consciousness is not this body, however, but the soul. The Nyayas believed in an infinite number of souls, one to each living organism. These souls are eternal and omnipresent; that is, each soul pervades the entire universe. It became necessary to postulate this as the soul had already been defined as illimitable. Though it pervades the entire universe, each soul is connected to only one consciousness, that of the particular living organism.

In Nyaya, the soul by itself is unthinking; all thought is derived from the mind, which is a part of the human body. The brain here is seen as a sort of machine only, processing all knowledge and relaying it to the soul, which gives the appearance of consciousness when these impressions are received. The intricate system of knowledge that Nyaya philosophers had developed showed that knowledge is something that is a part of human experience, and hence they were obliged to account for human knowledge within the human body. This led to a curious conclusion where the soul is seen as nothing more than a blank screen on which the mind relays its images and thus gives it its apprehension of consciousness. The soul has no inherent consciousness, giving rise to it only when it is in conjunction with the human mind.

Death is seen as merely the soul leaving its body. The soul then carries the impressions and weaknesses derived from its life cycle and accordingly takes up another body. This goes on until the soul lives such a perfect life that it is able to break through this cycle. In moksha the soul is no longer tied to consciousness and remains in its own eternal existence, unchanged and unruffled.

This metaphysical theory was weak on several points and was subjected to intense criticism by the other schools even when they accepted the Nyaya system of logic. In the first place, the concept of an infinite number of souls surviving eternally appears unsatisfactory, and how the souls relate to each other and to the material world is never explained. With each soul pervading every part of the universe, the universe too seems to be overcrowded with souls, with each point in space having a virtually infinite number of souls. The Nyaya view is essentially an atheistic one in which no god is recognized beyond this multiplicity of souls. In this case, it might be asked, who gave to them this law of karma whereby they are bound to rebirth until morality finally breaks the circle?

More difficult is the relation of the soul to consciousness. The soul by itself is unconsciousness, and consciousness is generated only when the soul is in conjunction with a mind. This makes the Nyayika view of moksha extremely unattractive, in which the soul shakes off its conscious impressions and returns to a state of unconsciousness. The soul is said to be in deep sleep when the mind stops relaying its images. A view of moksha that is not different from deep sleep can hardly be called an edifying one. Although there is no doubt that it is much sought after, hardly anyone would care to have a good sleep as his or her ideal afterlife!

However, the strength of the essence of the Nyaya system of logic is not to be doubted, and Nyaya terms used in arguments continue to be used today. Much of logic used thereafter in Indian philosophy was based on the Nyaya system.

The Vaisesika system is mainly analytical, and it seeks to determine the ultimate constituents of the world. In general it accepts the Nyayika theory of souls and God. In return, its atomistic explanation for the world is accepted by Nyaya. Just as the Nyayikas sought to understand knowledge—that is, what is inside our minds—by dissecting knowledge into its constituent parts or statements of logic and then examining them, the Vaisesikas sought to dissect the external world (i.e., the objects of the world) into its constituent parts and then study these parts to develop an understanding of them.

The theory of the Vaisesikas is the atomic theory. The Vaisesikas proposed that the universe comprises an infinite number of eternal and indivisible particles called atoms. These atoms combine with each other and produce the material world. The Vaisesikas developed their own system of classification of the substances of the world. The constituents of the world are divided into five categories: Akasa (space), earth, water, fire, and air. Each has their own distinguishing quality by which it appears as reality to the senses of ear, nose, tongue, eye, and skin. Akasa is distinguished by sound, air by tangibility, fire by color, water by taste, and earth by smell. Again, Akasa contains sound, air contains sound and tangibility, fire contains color along with sound and tangibility, water contains taste along with the preceding sensory inputs, and earth contains within it all the elements of smell, taste, color, tangibility, and sound. Thus the constituents of the world are related in a series to our sense organs. The elements are arranged in a sequence—Akasa, air, fire, water, and earth—and the evolution of these elements moves from the simple to the complex. That is, from Akasa arises air; from air, fire; from fire, water; and from water, earth.

These different qualities of the world derive from different atoms. The Vaisesikas recognized four different classes of atoms, each having their particular quality of earth, water, air, and fire. These four classes of atoms would aggregate in different proportions, thus giving to each object in nature different properties. Several such atoms combined to form the first visible particle, which was said to be the size of a speck in the sunlight. Since the atoms were individually without size, they needed to have an intermediary in order to combine. This was defined as Akasa, which is not strictly analogous to space. Akasa, which is not particulate either, holds the atoms together.

It is important to note that the five elements noted here are not accidental. Although humanity and everything in this world appears highly varied, all in reality comprise these same five elements.

Every particle in a human body and everything else in this world is made up of a mixture of elements derived from earth, water, and air; fire signifies the energy present in the body and Akasa the space that it occupies. Thus these five elements are both essential and also sufficient to constitute the human body.

The main contribution of the Vaisesikas was in the atomic theory of the constitution of matter. This appeared to be the first attempt by Hindu thinkers to deal with the physical world; otherwise it was the metaphysical implications of the internal world that involved them more. Latter-day Vaisesikas also seem to have anticipated a revolutionary view of our times. The further evolution of the material constitution of matter eventually led to problems in considering how space and time could be separately related to particles of matter, and latter-day Vaisesikas declared that space and time were one in reality, though conceived as twofold due to diverse effects. Latter Nyayikas described space and time as the modes of God. In their attempt to classify all of matter, they propounded the theory that all of matter was composed of name (the idea in our mind) and form (our sensory experience). This gave the term "nama-rupa" or "name-form" used always after that in Hinduism to describe the external world.

Like the Nyayikas, the Vaisesikas distinguished between matter and spirit and essentially held the same belief about the soul and its characteristics. Like the Nyayikas again, they had to face the same criticism about their metaphysics. The difficulties about the soul were the same. The atomic theory also had severe problems and was subjected to severe criticism by other schools of philosophy.

If the atoms do not have any size or dimension, it is difficult to see how they can carry qualities in themselves. Moreover, atoms of earth, for example, would have more qualities (four) then atoms of say, fire (two). Therefore, by any logic, they should be larger in size, yet all atoms are defined to be without any size. Again, how can atoms, which do not have size, aggregate together? Where would they touch with each other? If an individual atom does not have size, then an aggregate of atoms themselves would also not have size and remain infinitely small. Why in fact do the atoms aggregate together, as there is no god who directs them to do so and there is no individual will of the atoms themselves? The atoms by themselves are considered inactive, yet they must show activity in order to aggregate. These and similar arguments were faced by all atomic theorists, including the Greeks.

It is interesting to note that these two schools of Indian philosophy have much in common with Greek philosophy. The system of logic of the Nyayikas has much in common with the Aristotelian teachings. The atomic theory of the Vaisesikas again is very similar to Greek thought. This has resulted in the inevitable controversy whereby westerners declared that the Nyayikas derived their knowledge from the Greeks while Indians, as expected, say it was the opposite way. In this context, it is very significant that Pythagoras, to whom most of these Greek ideas can be traced, including those of Aristotle and Plato, has himself recounted that he visited India and derived much of his knowledge from there. But a close study of the history of the two philosophies shows that they are probably quite indigenous developments. Besides, there are small but important differences in the two systems. This makes it far more likely that the two systems developed independently, with perhaps some initial inputs from India to Greece.

This atomic theory dominated much of all metaphysical thinking, more so in the Greek and Western cultures than in India, where it was eventually defeated by more coherent philosophies. In fact, the atomic theory continues today even in modern science. The first scientific position of the indivisible atom was propounded by Dalton, which delighted the deterministic thought of the late-eighteenth century. But the atomic theory suffers from a fundamental flaw: it has to assume a smallest particle at one point, or else the theory will degenerate into eternal regression with smaller and smaller particles being proposed. In fact we see this happening today in quantum mechanics, where once the atom was discovered to have smaller subatomic particles, there has been a continuous finding of smaller and vaguer particles apparently into infinity. Efforts to put a stop to this by proposing a final "atom" such as the superstrings theory, will probably meet with the same failure as all previous atomic theories.

The Samkhya and Yoga Schools

The Purusha, the indwelling self, of the size of a thumb, is ever seated in the hearts of men. One should unerringly separate Him from one's body like a stalk from the munja grass. One should know Him as pure and immortal. Him one should know as pure and immortal.

—Katha Upanishad II.iii.17

The Samkhya school is believed to be the oldest school of philosophy in India, older even than the Vedanta. The school has as its fountainhead the mythical sage Kapila muni. To the muni is ascribed the book on Samkhya philosophy, Samkhya karika.

The Samkhya philosophy is important because, for the first time, it looks on the world as a whole. Other philosophers trying to understand the world, both internal and external, had divided everything into its constituent parts and tried to arrange them into different categories so as to analyze them separately. But this school looked at the whole world as a single entity; it "added" up different parts into a whole, and said that everything was part of a single reality. The goal then was to study this single, original entity, from which all others were derived.

From this thinking emerged an important idea that was to change the whole concept of metaphysics: the idea of evolution. The Samkhyas for the first time said that there was no omnipotent creator who created each part of the world separately and put them on the earth. Instead they advanced the idea of evolution, that the constituents of the world gradually evolved from each other, thus originally being part of each other. With the world being seen as a whole, the search now was for the essential unity. This idea of evolution was not scientific but philosophical and did not have the rationale of the Darwinian Theory. This was an evolution from spirits, the first being a principle called the *Mahat*, from which ultimately evolved the senses and finally the human.

The Samkhya idea of evolution extended further than the modern idea, as it encompassed the whole of the universe in its scope and said that the universe traveled in the cosmic cycle of evolution and involution. It also related human beings to the rest of the universe, both inanimate and animate. Humanity was seen not as a separate creation but as a part and only a further evolution of plants and animals. Life also was seen as not fundamentally different from non-life but only a further step on the path of evolution. The Samkhya evolution was also fundamentally different from modern evolution in that it proposed a direction, a goal for evolution. In Samkhya, all objects in the universe have a tendency to further evolve toward the goal of realization, and evolution takes place when obstacles to its path are removed. Thus even a rock can turn into a sage if the obstacles that are preventing it from doing so were to be removed. This idea was to be further developed in the Yoga system of Indian philosophy and influenced the whole of Indian philosophy, promising the goal of realization to all if only they were able through various means to remove the obstacles in their path.

The Samkhya idea of psychology is also interesting. Human consciousness is said to be constituted by three elements. The primary one that has cosmic significance is Buddhi, the intellect or the decision-making element of the mind. It works together with the Ahamkara or the ego, whose function is self-love. The Manas or mind is the organ that collects and makes sense of the impressions brought by the sense organs, and which suggests alternate courses of action. These are then presented to the Buddhi, which then along with the Ahamkara makes decisions. These three are the constituent parts of the internal organ of consciousness, the Antahkarna. Sometimes it is said they are the three modes of the Antahkarna.

The Samkhyas would have another important contribution to make in Indian philosophy. They also advanced the theory of the *gunas*, Sattva, Rajas, and Tamas. These were also present in the Vaisesika and Nyaya system, but it was here that the ideas were fully developed. In the Samkhya view, the gunas are the constituent strands of all matter. Sattva is the quality of lightness, of goodness; Rajas is the quality of activity and produces vitality; and Tamas is the quality of inertia and produces unhappiness. In later Vedanta, these qualities were seen more as the psychological trends of humans rather than in such cosmological terms of constituent strands of nature. These qualities were also found in the Nyaya and Vaisesika where they were seen as the qualities of nature and not constituent parts as such.

The Samkhya view of the metaphysical reality of the world is of the legendary duality, the *Purusha* and *Prakriti*, the male and the female principles. This was an idea that was to reverberate in philosophies and religions around the world. The Purusha, the male principle, is the eternal subject and the unmoving principle, whereas Prakriti, the female principle, is the eternal object and the creative principle.

The principle of Purusha-Prakriti is derived from the Samkhya view of cause and effect. In Samkhya, the effect exists beforehand in the cause. The effect is only an evolution of the cause and is not a new-formed thing. When milk (the cause, because it exists first) turns into curd (the effect, because it comes later), the curd already exists as a potential in the milk and it is manifested when under particular conditions such as heat, as the factors obstructing its manifestation are removed. All creation is only a development of the cause and all destruction is an envelopment into the cause. In any object, the past and future states of its existence are not destroyed and exist in it as potentialities that can be seen by Yogis.

For a cause to turn into effect—that is, its further stage of evo- lution—two factors are required: the material, for example, the milk, and the force that brings about the change, which is heat in this example. Everything in the world is related to its past in a cause and effect change. Again, nothing new can be created, as it would mean something produced from nothing. Hence the cause must contain at least as much if not more reality than its effect.

With this theorizing, the Samkhya asks, what is the cause of which all this is an effect? There must be a cause for everything, otherwise there would be a regression into infinity and this is not acceptable to Samkhya. The final cause must hence itself be an uncaused, that is, it itself would not be the effect of anything but would stand by itself. It would also contain in itself all reality that is seen in the present universe. The Samkhyas posit the duality of Purusha-Prakriti as this cause, Prakriti as the material aspect out of which all this universe is evolved and Purusha as the energy aspect that brings about this change in Prakriti.

The Purusha is the conscious, motionless, and the eternal knower whereas Prakriti is unconscious, active, constantly changing, and the eternal known. Prakriti is the creative principle in that it becomes changed into the created whereas Purusha remains unchanged but brings about the evolution in Prakriti. Prakriti is composed of three strands like that in a rope, the Sattva, Rajas, and Tamas. Before evolution, these three gunas are in perfect harmony and Prakriti is then in an unevolved stage. At the beginning of evolution, this harmony is disturbed by Purusha and the whole cycle begins. Purusha, the unmoving principle, does not actively cause this disturbance but its effect is said to be similar to the effect of a magnet on iron. Purusha sets Prakriti into motion rather like rolling a snowball down a hill would cause an avalanche.

Once Prakriti is set into motion it continues to evolve out into all the potentialities inherent in it. The internal organ of consciousness, the Antahkarna with its Buddhi, Manas, and Ahamkara, belongs to Prakriti and is by itself unconscious, merely registering these impressions. It is only when it comes into conjunction with the Purusha, which is inherently conscious, that the Antahkarna is illumined by consciousness. The Antahkarna reflects the Purusha like a reflection in a mirror and hence reflects its consciousness also and thus is invested with consciousness.

The Purusha remains eternally free, but when it is in conjunction with Prakriti, Prakriti casts its shadow on the Purusha and deludes it into thinking it is in bondage. The world is formed from this union of Purusha and Prakriti. When this union is broken, both Purusha and Prakriti are freed from this bondage and Purusha remains in eternal stability while Prakriti becomes once more harmonious in its three gunas. This is achieved through Yoga. The Samkhya theory is essentially atheistic as there is no room for God in this concept of duality.

The Samkhya theory of duality had a vital influence in the realm of Hindu thought and through it, in other parts of the world. The concept of male-female duality resurfaced time and again as the Shiva—Shakti duality with the Shaivaites worshipping the eternal and unchanging principle, Shiva, and the Shaktas (Tantra) worshipping the female creative principle, Shakti. It is also seen in Vaishnavism as the Krishna-Radha duality and in Chinese philosophy, to which it had spread through Buddhism, as the Yin-Yang concept.

Despite all its influence however, the Samkhya metaphysics had some fundamental weaknesses, which came under criticism from other schools. The concept of the individual Purusha is only slightly more advanced than the Nyaya-Vaisesika concept of the soul, with there being an infinite number of Purushas, which all exist coextensively. In Samkhya though, the Purusha has consciousness and is thus spared an eternity of sleep. The vital problem of all dualistic thought, how to relate the conscious with the unconscious, the Purusha with Prakriti, remains, with the union not being sufficiently explained. How and why Purusha combines with Prakriti, brings about its change, and then separates from it in moksha appears without any explanation whatsoever. Samkhya metaphysics eventually suffered a downfall, but its ideas remained as a vital stream of influence in Hinduism. It was only later that this concept of male-female duality was to achieve its sophistication in Shaivism and Tantra.

> *Saying "come, come," uttering pleasing words such as "this is your well earned virtuous path that leads to heaven," and offering him adoration, the scintillating oblations carry the sacrificer along the rays of the sun.*
>
> —Mundaka Upanishad I.ii.6

The Yoga school is considered as a part of the Yoga-Samkhya school as a whole. The Samkhya relates to the theoretical part of this school and Yoga to the practical side.

Yoga was established by the sage Patanjali in the Yoga sutras. It is concerned with the individual's path to realization. The Samkhya had laid down in theory the belief that superhuman powers and, eventually, realization could be achieved by all and was already present in potential in all of us. The Yogic school developed a detailed path toward realizing this dream. The path of Yoga was through the use of the mind, using concentration to heighten our power over the mind and thus to conquer it. This enables us to go beyond the limits of ordinary human activities and achieve a higher level of existence. Realization can be achieved by suppressing the mind totally so that the soul remains in a state of tranquility and bliss.

The Yoga system for the first time spoke of a fundamental axiom that had tremendous influence in religion: the supremacy of mind over matter. The highest form of matter in Yoga was the *chitta*, the mind substance, the material out of which the mind is made. This was actually a part of matter, and hence it could be used to dominate over all matter. Because we could learn to control the mind, in effect we could dominate over all matter. Yoga also in its path exalted silence and solitude, meditation and indifference to outer conditions and material life. This influenced and changed all of Hindu religious life and continues to characterize the Hindu in the eyes of the outer world.

The Yoga system accepts without any qualifications the Samkhya view of metaphysics. It only makes one important change, the addition of God in the Samkhya scheme of things. The God of Yoga is a personal god, and he initiates creation at the outset from Prakriti by enjoining Purush to Prakriti. He also gives the law of karma to the souls and ensures its functioning. As has been pointed out, there is little other function of God besides this and the conception of God seems almost superfluous in Yoga. It was perhaps only a historical bow to the rising tide of theism. Also, Yogic teachers perhaps recognized the power of a spiritual force directed toward a higher being in which the aspirant could repose full faith, and it was to harness this force that God was created as a concept.

The other important change that Yoga makes is in the sphere of psychology. The later Samkhya texts had already indicated that the three organs of consciousness, namely intellect or Buddhi, mind or Manas, and ego or Ahamkara, were but three modifications of the internal organ, the Antahkarna. Yoga, with its great stress on psychology, finally declared that all three are one and only modifications of what it called chitta, the mind substance. All impulses in the mind are like vibrations in this chitta. Intellect, ego, and mind are parts of this same chitta. Chitta is in a contracted state when it is associated with a lower being, such as an animal, and expanded in a being such as a human. In its highest state, in the unevolved state, it is all-pervading. The aim of Yoga is to control this chitta by controlling and suppressing its vibrations and thus reach its all-pervading state. The Purusha associated with that chitta then becomes free. Chitta by itself is unconscious and is lit by consciousness by the Purusha. After making these changes in its metaphysics to correspond with its practices, Yoga goes on to outline the method of practice.

The importance of the Yogic school to Hinduism can hardly be overemphasized, even though its metaphysics would eventually be surrendered. Hindu religious practice since then is based mainly on the Yogic precepts.

By far the most important book of Yoga philosophy is the Yoga Sutras by Patanjali. This ancient book has an all-pervading influence over Hinduism through the method of Yoga that it taught. Although Yoga has continued to develop throughout the ages, this book was the "primer" upon which all the systems of Yoga are based. Patanjali outlined eight steps of Yoga, from the dos and don'ts of social life to the last step of mystical union with the absolute. The main system of Yoga taught in these sutras is Jnana Yoga, the Yoga of knowledge, in which the goal is sought through the mind by using the method of meditation. But the eight steps serve as guidelines for all the systems of Yoga. Thus, even though the philosophy of the Yoga system was submerged by superior forms, its teachings continue to shape the practice of all Hindu systems.

The Purva Mimamsa School

The Purva Mimamsa school is based on a very literal and dogmatic interpretation of the Vedas. It takes as given all arguments and injunctions given in the Vedas and concerns itself only with the implementation of these injunctions.

The Vedas, as we have seen, contain four parts: the Samhita, Brahmana, Aranyaka, and Upanishads. The Samhita part consists of hymns, which are addressed to various gods, mainly to Indra, the king of gods, and also to other deities like Agni (fire) and Usha (the dawn). In these hymns the deities are praised and *Yagnas*, or ritual worship ceremonies to these deities, are referred to. The hymns describe these rituals only very sketchily.

The next section of the Vedas, the Brahmanas, are completely devoted to these rituals or Yagnas, and it is this section that is the main subject of the Purva Mimamsa. The Yagnas differ in their complexity and the largest ones may go on up to a year and requiring the involvement of mind boggling details and objects of worship. To some extent, these Yagnas survive in modern Hinduism in the household *pujas* and ceremonies connected to marriage, death, and birth in Hindu life. These Yagnas in the main consist of an altar containing fire into which the specially trained priests pour various offerings to the accompaniment of chanted mantras. The benefit of the Yagna goes to the householder who organizes these Yagnas. Many of these Yagnas involve sacrifice of animals, with some of the Tantric cults involving even sacrifice of human beings, although this would never have been accepted in the Vedas or mainstream Hinduism. The Brahmanas give all details of these sacrifices including the shape and size of the fire altar, the number of priests and the mantras each have to chant, the objects to be offered to the fire, the timing of the Yagna, and so forth.

The Yagnas are timed according to the lunar calendar and depend on the position of the planets. This necessitated a very detailed knowledge of planetary movements, which are still followed in Hindu almanacs called *Panjika*, one of which is to be found in practically every Hindu household. It is a vital part of most Hindu households, as things like pujas and ceremonies have to be timed according to this. The level of astronomical knowledge is astounding, and illiterate Indians from all over the country will gather at special sites on certain astronomical events like solar eclipses at the precise date and time that has been predicted as accurately by their ancient texts as any modern astronomical almanac. An interesting aspect of these Yagnas is that, for the householders, both husband and wife are required to be present and to participate jointly; each is considered incomplete without the other. The Brahmanas give details of the deities that are to be propitiated at different times and the benefits that the Yagna will bring to the householders.

Besides the large Yagnas, the Vedas and its subsidiary texts also describe many smaller rituals that are to be observed at different times, like prayers to be said at dawn and at evening, during baths, during the change of the seasons, during full and new moons, and for many more occasions. The texts also describe the foods to eat, how to cook the food, the duties of each man and woman, and so forth. It is in these texts—both in the Vedas and the subsidiary texts—that the strict caste laws of Hindu society are laid down. The observation of all these laws and countless rituals is considered mandatory and leads one to heaven.

The Purva Mimamsa concerns itself mainly with this ritualistic observation of the Vedas. The Vedas are considered eternal, not just in the sense that the truths preached by them are eternal, but in the sense that the words of the Vedas themselves are eternal. The *rishis* or seers who composed them only heard these words in meditation and brought them to the attention of humanity, but the words themselves had always existed. Not even God is granted the authorship of the Vedas, the Vedas themselves are "God" in Purva Mimamsa.

As the school of Purva Mimamsa bases itself on the truth of words, an elaborate theory of words was established in order to uphold their theory. In Purva Mimamsa there is an eternal relation between a word and the object it denotes. Words were not created by the human race but were merely uttered for the first time, having already existed in eternity. If one does not recognize a word, it does not mean that the relationship of the word to the object is not present, but merely that we do not have the knowledge of the relation. Words do not change; they are only replaced by new words. Words have naturally denotative powers whether we understand their meanings or not. Thus human languages were not "invented" but "discovered," and the words of these languages existed prior to humans and will live on even if the human race dies out.

While at first glance the Mimamsa theory on words might seem a bit far-fetched, it has exerted a very strong influence in diverse fields. The importance of mantras in both Hindu and Buddhist Tantras and the repetitive chanting of a certain word or a very short prayer by mystics in Christianity and Islam depend on similar theories. A similar idea was also expressed in the Biblical words, "In the beginning was the Word. . . ." Modern grammar theoreticians also emphasize an inherent relation between words and their meanings for us; we cannot conceive of any thought without words, hence all our thoughts and therefore virtually everything within us depends solely on words. The relation between a word and its meaning is therefore a given relation, which is not debatable by logic.

The other great importance of Mimamsakas was in Hindu law. The Mimamsakas were the main guardians of laws in the Vedas and their subsidiary texts, and their interpretations were accepted by all other schools. Even modern Hindu laws in the Indian constitution depend to a large extent on their interpretations. Much of Hindu society even today continues to be governed by the edicts set down in the Vedic scriptures, and to the Mimamsa goes the responsibility of transmission of all these Vedic traditions, both the evils (such as the caste system), as well as the good (such as its tolerance, strong faith, and spiritual freedom).

With their implicit belief in the words of the Vedas, the teachers of Purva Mimamsa did not need to concern themselves with the ideas behind words. It was enough that certain injunctions were given in the Vedas promising certain benefits. Hence there was very little metaphysical thought in this school. They accepted without hesitation the different deities given in the Vedas to whom the Yagnas were devoted. There was no all-powerful God in Mimamsa, although it was introduced in later writings. Since the Vedas promised a heaven in the afterlife, having a soul became necessary to enjoy that life, but there was very little speculation regarding the soul and its relationship with the rest of the system. Such an empty ritualistic religion could not satisfy most people, and the Purva Mimamsa exerted its hold only on the dogmatic sections of society, becoming the strongest when Hindu society turned inward-looking. In the face of more vigorous and spiritually satisfying thought, the Mimamsa survived only on the fringes of religious paths, although its influence has continued in other ways.

The Vedantic School

It is in the Vedantic (*aant* means "end," hence *Vedantic* is the end part of the Vedas) or *Upanishadic* school where for the first time we have the concept of a *single* truth beyond this world. In Nyaya-Vaisesika, the higher truth was a complex of souls and atoms. In Samkhya and Yoga, the higher truth was the duality of Purusha-Prakriti. In Purva Mimamsa, the higher truth comprised a galaxy of gods and goddesses who ruled over the world. But in the Upanishads, we find the concept of a single higher truth.

This higher truth of the Upanishads is the Brahman. It is here that we see a concept of religion that would be recognizable outside India, where religion usually means a theistic religion—that is, one that accepts a single, higher truth. The relationship of Brahman to the world is interpreted in three major ways, which are basically the three ways of all theism. The three ways are the dualistic, qualified monistic, and monism or Advaita.

Dualism

Where are they now today? Where art thou, the Gods in heaven?
Who is the man ye strive to reach? Who of your supplicants
* is with you?*
Whom do ye visit, whom approach? To whom direct your
* harnessed car?*
With whose devotions are ye pleased? We long for you to further us.
—Rig Veda 5.74

The most famous of the dualistic interpreters of the Upanishads was Madhava. Like other scholars of the Vedantas, he concentrated more on the Brahma Sutras than the Upanishads, although he commented on a number of Upanishads also.

Madhava recognized three classes of existence. In fact all dualists, despite being called so, recognize these three classes. They are

God, the soul, and the substance or matter of the universe. Madhava made it clear that all three are distinct and separate from each other. Life or consciousness is connected only with the soul, the matter of the universe is unconscious, and God is super-conscious. The life of a human is connected with the soul he or she possesses; the body itself is unconscious. God is beyond everything; his ways are beyond human understanding. God has created these two classes of existence for his own purposes and created them merely by his wish practically out of nothing.

The Christian and Islamic orthodox views are also dualistic worldviews. In the Bible, God created the entire universe in six days by uttering a word, which would make the thing materialize (another instance of an eternal relation between the word and the object it denotes). Humans were created on the last day and God breathed life into the body, that is, gave them a soul. Thus the three classes of existence and their eternal differences are defined in the myth of creation. The Islamic view is similar with Allah creating humans out of clay and then giving them life.

There are many objections to such dualistic beliefs. The simplest one asks why we should believe in such stories. There is no logical basis for belief in such a God. The commonest reason given for such beliefs is the incredible beauty and variety of life, and it is said that such richness necessarily needs a higher power, someone with supernatural qualities to have conceived and created all this. This of course flies against the knowledge that we have today, as we now know that this was created by nature itself through evolution, and it is the struggle of life against all odds that has given rise to its beauty. Besides, although there is beauty, there is great destruction in nature as well. Although we might see the wonders of the human body, we also have to contend with the numerous illnesses and handicaps that befall us. A similar feeling of awe arises when we contemplate nature in its macroscopic grandness as well, as when we wonder at the stars and the vastness of space. But as physics probes further into space, this too is seen to have a rationale existence and in fact all types of questions are now raised that make this vast space seem totally unlike what we conceive it to be.

The complexity of human life and its apparent futility when it all ends in death is another reason given, as it is said there must be a higher reason for this and someone must have a plan for all this. This again goes against reason, as we might well suppose that life is indeed futile; the despair that this might give rise to is not reason enough to posit a grand conception of god as a cover. Besides, other religions might well have found a different explanation that makes life livable. Religions like Buddhism and Advaitism do not need a concept of a creator god to give harmony to life. Another reason given is that so many people have believed in this, hence it must be true. This also cannot be accepted just as we cannot accept that the earth is flat just because so many people once believed it to be so.

Another reason preached so commonly, that we should accept God because it is written in a particular book or because some great man preached about it many years ago, is asking almost too much from any person with modern views, requiring him or her to give up all belief in science and our modern way of thought. The huge advancements of science have had a corrosive effect on dualistic beliefs, squeezing the rationale of belief in such gods further and further.

An important argument against such a personal God is why God should have created us all in the first place, if it was just to put us in a testing ground in which he controls all the sides and decides the handicaps, and then judge us and give us heaven or hell. It seems an utterly pointless thing to do, especially when we consider all the suffering and injustice that so many have to go through. Saying he does it for his play or amusement is hardly satisfying; in fact it would make us quite indignant to think of God chortling away in his heaven even as he makes someone's life particularly wretched or deals out large-scale disasters. Saying his purposes are beyond human understanding is only an evasion of an answer. Also, if he did create the universe out of his will, then it means even he has desires and is therefore not all-powerful; he might well have many other desires besides.

There are a whole range of other questions that dualism by and large ignores, although a more discerning mind can hardly refrain from asking them. Dualism ignores questions like how the conscious mind controls the unconscious body, all problems connected with the concept of a soul, such as whether we may consider viruses to have souls and such other things, the question of the relativity and hence lack of absolute reality of the universe, and more.

In spite of all their difficulties, dualistic beliefs are held by a very large number of people. This is mainly due to force of habit among people who have not clearly examined their beliefs or asked themselves enough questions. Besides, the strength and power given by such beliefs cannot be ignored. The simple knowledge that there is a God who loves us and who has a higher purpose for us gives more satisfaction and strength than all the scientific and philosophical knowledge put together. It is in this appeal to the heart in which the strength of dualism lies, and mere intellectual questioning cannot dispel such beliefs. The richness of such beliefs must be respected and their strength and inspiration are resources from which no human heart can afford to be cut off completely.

Qualified Monism

Qualified monism holds that the world is a changed or qualified form of God. Qualified monism, in examining the relationship between God and the world, differs from dualism in that it declares that God and this world are not two completely different entities; rather, it says that the world is a part of God. The world itself is considered to be divine and worthy of worship or knowledge. The vital difference with dualism is that here there is no absolute difference between the world and God; the world is a part of God and God is immanent or "dissolved" in the world, so that everything here is ultimately a "qualified" state of God, and hence divine. Qualified monists find the divine here within this life, and try to merge into this divinity. Qualified monism says that all things that are seen in the world are but different forms of the same single state or form of existence. This existence is changed or qualified into the various objects and phenomena of the world, hence the term "qualified monism." This Reality, of which the world is a part, is the goal of spiritual quest in qualified monism.

Again, qualified monism differs from Advaitism or monism in that it recognizes the reality of the world and says that God, or the absolute, and the world are equally real—that is, God (or rather, a part of God) is really changed into the Universe (unlike in Advaitism where the change is not considered a "real" change). In Advaitism, the world is manifested from the absolute, but because it is of relative reality only, the only reality that exists is that of the absolute. But in qualified monism, the world is considered to have equal reality with the absolute; hence it exists and is of a permanent nature. This means that the world is not the absolute itself but has its own identity, its own existence in itself. Hence the world and the absolute both exist as two entities, with the world being a lower part of the absolute, or God.

Qualified monism is thus a halfway house between dualism and Advaitism. It does not accept the complete difference between God and the world as in dualism nor does it accept, as in monism or Advaitism, that the world has only relative reality and the only reality is the absolute.

Besides the difference in the philosophy of metaphysics, these differences are most important for spiritual practice. Unlike in dualism, in qualified monism the world, and humanity, enjoys a far more exalted position. We are not completely separate from the Lord; we all carry within ourselves a spark from God. There is thus a divinity within us; we are all part of the divine. Hence qualified monism is a far more harmonious and softer form of religion than pure orthodox dualism. Dualistic concepts like original sin, fire and brimstone hells, and so on would not apply in qualified monism. It brings humankind much nearer to God than dualism.

Again, qualified monism differs from Advaitism or monism because it recognizes the ultimate reality of our personal consciousness. Qualified monism recognizes the reality of both the absolute consciousness and the individualized consciousness. But in Advaitism it is not our personal identity that is true, but only our absolute identity, Brahman. This means that we are in essence already God, already the absolute. In Qualified monism, there is not a complete merger of the soul with God in mysticism, as the soul is considered as only a "part" of God, and hence a difference always remains. But in Advaitism, there is no true reality of the individual consciousness, and we ourselves are the absolute in all its reality; hence, a state is attained in which there is no difference whatsoever from the absolute.

Advaitic practices consist of trying to annihilate our individual consciousness so that the absolute alone remains, while in qualified monism the individual consciousness attempts to approach nearer to God. In Advaitism we can say, I am the absolute, Ahm Brahmasi. The absolute then is not something that is above us; it is I myself. God then is no longer a supreme, benevolent being who rules over us and we do not have anymore a god to pray to or to beseech, to blame for our sorrows and thank for our happiness. So the concept of a personal god is lost. But in qualified monism, God is a supreme higher principle of which the world is only a part, and hence there is a personal god to pray to.

The qualified monistic interpretation of the Vedantas rose out of opposition to Shankara's tradition of monism, which was mainly intellectual. It was spearheaded by Ramanuja, who passionately attacked Advaitism for its cold logic and preached a qualified monistic theory, which allowed for a more emotional interpretation of the relation between God and humans.

The doctrine of Ramanuja is the main form of Vedantic qualified monism. In Ramanuja's religion, the one reality is considered to be a God with will, and all the world is considered to be the body of this God. Qualified monism of Ramanuja recognizes three existences—God, soul, and matter—but unlike dualism, it says the latter two were created both by and out of God, and hence God and the world are not two fundamentally different entities. Our souls are like sparks from the fire, which is God; the world is like a spider's web, which it weaves by extruding it from its own body. Hence there is a divine basis of both our souls and all of the universe, because the base material out of which we are composed is God. We are ultimately a part of God, and God is a part of us. God is present within us and within every living thing, and he is also immanent in the world. We need not look for God outside, as in dualism, but can find Him in ourselves. God created us by his own free will and started off the whole cycle of reincarnation. In other respects, Ramanuja also accepts the theory of reincarnation with the same cycle of rebirth, heaven, and finally moksha. But unlike in the dualistic view, moksha is not simply nearness to God but actual contact. Here the soul retains its identity but remains in touch with God, and hence is able to share in the divine bliss of God.

Many beautiful analogies are used to describe the relationship between human souls and God in qualified monism. Analogies like the fire and spark, the pot and the earth, and jewelry and gold are some of the ones used in the Upanishads. In all these, there is a base material, earth, sea, or gold, out of which is created a form, such as the pot, wave, or jewelry. This form then acquires a name. Thus all things in this world are but different forms and names of the same base material, God. Another analogy used in qualified monism is that of the cells and the human organism. We each have billions of cells within us and they are all living bodies in their own rights, including the brain cells. Similarly, we may all consider ourselves as cells of some higher organism, such as God. Just as an individual cell in our body would have no idea at all that it is part of a higher organism, so also do we not have an idea that we are a part of God, yet we fulfill some function of him. A similar analogy is that of the tree and its leaves.

Qualified monism is the most widespread position in Hinduism, being the main position of the Bhakti cults. Ramanuja gave a great impetus to the spread of Bhakti Yoga by defining a position that allowed one to have faith, and at the same time strength. A dualistic position is weakening, as it means that man must always be a servant of God. A monist position, on the other hand, has little appeal for the heart as it negates the concept of a God who is interested in us and who will help us. Qualified monism appeals to our senses because it accepts a God above us and at the same time speaks of a complete harmony in all, from all of nature to us and to God. Unlike Advaitism or Buddhism, it does not dismiss the world as a relative reality and accepts it as real, because it is a part of God. The ennobling influence of Bhakti spread rapidly, and today it may be said that the vast majority of Hindus in India are qualified monists rather than dualists. Most accept the doctrine of a "spark of divinity" existing within everything, as well as the need to search for God within ourselves rather than without. This is true even though most Hindus will participate in dualistic rituals with full vigor, because Bhakti has always recognized the importance of ritualism in the growth of spirituality.

Qualified monism has also led to the worship of nature in Hinduism. Since God is within everything, everything is God. Hence Hindus have numerous articles of nature, which are considered holy and are worshipped, mainly to access the inspiration of the divinity within. Thus there are holy rivers, cities, flowers, trees, animals, in fact virtually no end to holy objects. But the real worship is of a higher nature and has a deeper meaning than simple nature worship.

The main difficulty of qualified monism of Ramanuja, as with all qualified monism, is that it is a halfway house between dualism and monism, and its followers have to always be careful that they define themselves against the two ends of these beliefs.

Ramanuja accepts a God with a divine will who has created the world and humans out of his own will. In this he resembles dualism by defining a personal God who is omnipotent and inexplicable and rules over us all. But when he approaches too close to dualism, Ramanuja veers toward monism and says that God created humans and the world from his own substance and hence they are essentially all the same. Being a part of God means the absolute differences between the three substances (God, man, and matter) become blurred, and hence it brings the concept closer to monism. Again, to save himself from merger with monism, he says that the change is real and absolute, that man and matter are changed parts of God.

There is no firm dividing line between Advaitism and qualified monism. Both recognize a higher plane of existence, the absolute, and a lower plane, the world. The difference is whether we regard the world to be real or unreal; the more we accept the world as real, the more we go toward qualified monism, and the more we take it as unreal, the more we go toward Advaitism. Advaitism regards the world as only a "half-baked" reality and rejects it, instead accepting Brahman as the only true reality of everything in this world, including our individuality, whereas in qualified monism, both are equally real.

On the other side, after taking the world as real (which is the "middle" qualified monistic position) the more we emphasize the difference between the world and the absolute, the more we tend toward dualism. Qualified monists have to maintain their position by veering toward dualism when questioned by monism and toward monism when questioned by dualists. It is not a true position, and they survive by not following their arguments to their logical end, as they would then arrive at either dualism or monism.

Besides Ramanuja, other forms of qualified monism—both in Hinduism and in other religions like Christianity and Islam—all maintain their position at various points in between dualism and monism, being closer to one or the other. Ramanuja has been careful to stand in the middle.

Like dualism, qualified monism is ultimately a doctrinal position, and depends on entities defined by books or teachers. Its principles are not derived from the rigorous application of logic and reason to the world around us, as in Advaitism and Buddhism. Instead they depend on particular doctrines and scriptures, and call for our belief in them. Because of this, qualified monism is not a single position but has several variations, depending on the particular teaching, and there is also wide variation among different teachers within the same creed. Of course, qualified monism has also now been contradicted by modern science, which supports the view of the world not having any absolute reality.

> *O Thou who art the nourisher, the solitary traveler, the controller, the acquirer, the son of Prajapati, do remove thy rays, do gather up thy dazzle. I shall behold by thy grace that form of thine which is most benign. I am that very person who is yonder in the sun.*
>
> —Isa Upanishad XVI

Jainism, Taoism, and modern pantheism may also be considered to be forms of qualified monism. In these philosophies the world is considered to be a real, self-existing entity. But there is a vital difference with qualified monism as such because here there is no higher absolute or God. The world exists alone, there is no other entity than the world, and the world in its multi-dimensioned reality is the sole existence. Thus it differs from dualism, quali-fied monism, and Advaitism because it does not accept a higher absolute.

In Buddhism, also, there is no other entity than this world. But pantheism, Jainism, and Taoism differ fundamentally from Bud-dhism in that they recognize the world to have complete reality; the world is real in itself and there is no other reality apart from this world. But in Buddhism, the world is considered to be only relative reality, and the quest of spirituality is to achieve a higher realty than this world. Thus the spiritual goal is different from Buddhism.

The Jain religion in India arose concurrently with Buddhism. Its founder, Mahavira, was contemporary with Gautama Buddha. The Jains recognize the reality of the world and do not accept an absolute beyond this world. The Jain view of metaphysics is that the world is "permanent-in-change," or that the world is continuously chang-ing and hence there is nothing in it that has any permanent truth. The Jains accept an eternal and real existence, but they say the world is infinitely dimensioned and the reality that we see is only a very small part of the actual reality. Whatever knowledge we have of the world is also very limited, because it is only a small part of the actual reality. The true reality is the sum of all the forms that we see in the universe around us, and is infinitely larger and more multi-dimensioned than any individual existence.

Thus Jains accept the relation of parts and whole in respect to the world and the reality, as in cells to the human body or leaves to the tree. This all-encompassing reality is not a God with a will or a personal God but simply the sum of all the individual parts of the universe. There is no way that a person can ordinarily come to have knowledge of this whole complex reality. In the Jain view, everything exists in pairs, truth and untruth, good and bad, and they are both only a small aspect of the actual reality. Jainism also recognizes the existence of souls, but accepts a strict division between the soul and matter. The soul too is a form of existence of the whole reality, just as the body or other matter, but the soul is the highest state of existence.

Like all forms of qualified monism, Jainism too developed nature worship as a religious goal. But in Jainism, this nature worship reached its greatest extreme. All life is sacred in Jainism according to their teachings, and hence no life can be harmed. Strict Jain monks will cover their mouths while speaking, to prevent injuring any small organisms, which might enter their mouths. They also sweep the floor before them while walking for the same reason, and use only water that has been used for cooking by someone else; thus they can be sure that they will not be injuring any life themselves, as such water will already be free of life-forms. Jain monks also follow a very strict asceticism, and the highest monks do not wear any clothes at all, which, as may be understood, often causes quite a stir among conservative Hindus.

Jainism is also characterized by one of the most progressive codes of morality. The most important contribution of Jainism to the world is the idea of *ahimsa*, or nonviolence. The Jains practice ahimsa not just in deeds but in speech and thought also. Kindness to all forms of life is an integral part of the religion. Great emphasis is also placed on truth, renunciation, charity, etc. Along with this, there is a healthy regard for earning wealth, as this is necessary for the general members of the community in order to maintain the religion.

Like the Buddhists, the Jains have as their mystical goal the acquiring of the knowledge of reality in all its aspects, and not just the finite aspect that is known by an ordinary individual. It differs vitally from Buddhism in that it accepts this multifarious universe as the true reality, and seeks only to know it as real, unlike the Buddhists who consider this universe as unreal and try to know it as such, and strike it down, so that they can be free of it and attain nirvana. The Jains seek to achieve this by a program of ascetic practices like fasting and praying, and by meditation. Once this knowledge is attained, the person is freed from hankering for life and is then not reborn again.

But this form of mysticism has its inherent difficulties. The question arises that if there is no higher state of existence, if this is all, if even in moksha the best that is attained is that we are not reborn again, then what is the purpose of living? We may as well lie down and die. In fact in Jainism, which follows all doctrines to its logical extreme, this is the highest goal of all. This end is known in Jainism as Kaivalya, the equivalent of nirvana, and the highly developed monk attains it by simply refusing to take any food or drink until he or she gives up her life and attains this blessed oblivion. Such a religious practice hardly seems the answer to our spiritual quest.

Like other forms of qualified monism, Jains also found it difficult to maintain their position logically. Because the phenomena of the world are real, then behind different phenomena like a candle, wax, and smoke there must be a common base. Again, once this base is accepted, it has to be something, which is the basis for all phenomena. Arguing in this way, the Jains would ultimately arrive at a theory of a common absolute beyond all phenomena, instead of a multifaceted universe. Thus Jains, if they follow their logic strictly, end up in Advaitism, and many Jain scholars upheld a position that was indistinguishable from Advaitism. Hence, to delineate their religion, Jain texts had to maintain a strictly doctrinal definition. But despite some inherent contradictions, Jainism has had an important role to play in India, and its religious ideals have been accepted and respected throughout the country even by those of other religions.

Taoism, the religion of China, accepts the same basic reality of the world as Jainism. Its important belief is in the principle of Tao. Tao is the force that guides the fundamental rhythm of the universe. Taoism believes that the universe moves in a rhythmic cycle, and the principle of Tao is the driving force of this cycle. This cycle connects everything in the world, and the goal of spirituality is to move with this Tao, to let the Tao flow through us and thus achieve harmony with the universe. Meditation, calmness, prayers, and devotion to one's duty are the basic guiding principles of this path.

A similar philosophy is modern pantheism. This was the guiding philosophy of scientific thought, especially in the Newtonian age. Here also, the universe is considered to be the only reality and there is no other higher entity, but it does not accept any religious overtones and its quest is to know more of this reality through scientific exploration. However, with the realization that everything in the world has only relative reality, the confidence of being satisfied with knowing this universe alone has weakened, and modern spirituality must consider the question as to whether there is a higher reality that is beyond this world and to which we can aspire.

In Christianity and Islam also, we can see these three main forms of metaphysics, the dualistic, qualified monistic, and monistic. Jesus taught these three forms to his followers. Swami Vivekananda perceived them as being meant for different levels of followers according to their capacity. The first teaching of Jesus was, "I am the Son of God." This is the dualistic teaching, where there is a clear distinction between God and humans and God is a father figure who is controlling us all. The next teaching was, "the Father is in me and I am in the Father"; this is the qualified monistic teaching, where the spark of divinity is in each of God and us is immanent in us. The farthest teaching was, "I and the Father are one." This is the monistic teaching, where there is no longer any difference between God and humanity and a complete identity is preached.

In the early historical development of Christianity, all these three forms appear to have enjoyed equal importance and they developed side by side. This is still seen in the Asiatic form of Christianity. But in the Western world, gradually the dualistic form came to predominate and the orthodoxy tried to suppress other forms. But qualified and absolute monism continues to thrive in the teachings of the mystics of Christianity.

In Islam also, all these three forms can be easily discerned. The teaching of the Qu'ran is essentially a dualistic teaching. But with the Sufi mystics, we see the development of qualified monism and ultimately a monistic form of metaphysics. Here, too, although only the dualistic form is advanced by the orthodoxy, the other forms still retain their firm hold over their followers.

The Buddhist Position

Long is the night to him who is awake; long is a mile to him who is tired; long is life to the foolish who do not know the true law.

—Dhammapada 60

Buddhism was the religion propounded by Lord Gautama Buddha in the sixth century BCE. The story of Buddha is a noble one and shows his great love for people. All his sutras have one purpose, to help people in their lives in this world. The story is told of how Gautama Buddha was raised into awareness of human misery by the sight of four scenes: an old man, a sick man, a corpse, and a monk. Following this, he gave up his princely life and retired into the forests, where he attained realization and then began to preach his path of salvation for humanity.

Buddhism is based on the four great truths realized by the Buddha during intense meditation. Of these, the most important, the defining truth of Buddhism, is that the world is *dukha*, or suffering. The world—that is, human life—is filled with suffering and misery. Buddha then sets out to find how this can be remedied. The other truths proclaim that the cause of this misery is desire, that misery can be got rid of, and that the way to get rid of this misery is by following the eightfold path. The eightfold path in turn contains eight rules for our lives, such as right living, right thinking, avoiding lust, and more, including right meditation. By following these laws, one can get rid of misery and thus have a healthy life. The laws are similar to the commandments of Christianity and are a sort of rulebook of ethics aimed at giving Buddhists a clean, tranquil life. The simplicity of Buddha's teachings, his compassion, and his greatness captivated India, and for many centuries after his birth Buddhism became the state religion and the religion of the majority, supplanting Hinduism.

The path shown by Buddha was aimed at the salvation of humanity. Its end was a practical end, to enable people to attain peace and tranquility and resolve the problem of how best to live their lives. The religion of Buddha was not concerned with intricate metaphysical speculation. Buddha called his way the middle path. It was a path that avoided both asceticism and also the complex ritualism that was being practiced at that time. Instead, Buddha showed how spiritual goals could be achieved through simplicity, without taking recourse to either of these ways. Buddhism was also the "middle way" in that it was equidistant from the positions of absolutism or eternalism of Advaita and the nihilism of some Hindu schools.

That things die is proof that there is no eternalism. That things are born is proof that there is no nihilism. Buddha described the world as *anatta*, or non-self. If there is an absolute beyond this world, then there would be a ground of existence beyond everything in this world and hence beyond dukha also. This would mean that dukha would continue to exist in that ground and that it could not be got rid of completely. Thus the idea of an absolute leads to eternalism, an eternity of existence, and is hence rejected by Buddhism.

At the same time, Buddha also did not accept nihilism. The world could not be said to be nonexistent either. Hence Buddha postulated a position that lay between absolutism and nihilism. But Buddha refused to clearly define a metaphysical stand. He wanted to preach a religion that would be a help to humans in living their lives; therefore, he preached a system of values that would lead to a clean, simple life. He wanted to create a system of ethics that was not based on perilous metaphysical beliefs but that was based on this world itself. It was a system of beliefs that depended on humanity, not on supra-human powers or principles. Such a system did not need metaphysical speculation; in fact, Buddha declared that metaphysical speculation is an impediment to our spiritual path. Buddha gave the metaphor of the man who has an arrow in his chest. His requirement now is not to know who shot the arrow or what it was made of; his sole aim now would be to get the arrow out. Similarly, we all have the arrow of dukha in our hearts, and the aim is to get out of this dukha by following the eightfold path and not to indulge in metaphysical speculation.

Hence, because it was unnecessary, Buddha prescribed a rigid agnostic position by prohibiting metaphysical speculation. These are the sixty-two banned questions of Buddhism, which relate to metaphysics, such as whether the soul exists or not, whether the universe exists or not, and so on, and the Buddha simply refused to give an answer and in fact forbade these questions being raised. An interesting story is told of how, when the Buddha was asked whether there really was a God, he picked up a few dry leaves from the forest floor and said, "there are as many truths as the leaves of these forests, out of these I have held up only a few to you."

But such a doctrinal agnostic position could be accepted only by the most faithful of devotees. An agnostic position cannot satisfy the thirst for spirituality for most followers, and enquiring minds are bound to raise questions. Especially in a country like India, philosophical speculation is the lifeblood of any religion, and those with a more critical attitude demanded clear and specific answers to the important questions.

The Buddha consciously refrained from metaphysical speculation, but he had set the Buddhist position between the absolutism of Advaita and nihilism by rejecting both. The first truth discovered by Buddha stated that dukha, or this world, existed, and the third stated that dukha was not permanent. Buddhist philosophers now began to clearly define and defend this metaphysical stand. Thus almost from Buddha's death, various Buddhist scholars began giving arguments to buttress the Buddhist position. But soon major schisms developed among Buddhist scholars, and ultimately Buddhist metaphysics was divided into two schools: the Theravada or Hinayana, which is considered the original Buddhist position, and the Buddhism of the Sanskrit schools, Mahayana Buddhism.

Theravada Buddhism, like Advaitism, follows realistic metaphysics. Prior to beginning any metaphysical speculation, it accepts as existing on the same level of reality the trio of thinker, thought, and the thing thought of. Also like Advaitism, it believes that the existence of both the subject (the individual consciousness) and the object (the world outside) are a fuzzy existence, and that they have only relative reality and not absolute reality. But unlike Advaitism, Theravada Buddhism does not accept the presence of an absolute behind this relative existence and says it exists in itself. Beyond this there is nothing, and the world has only anatta, or non-self, as the basis.

Mahayana Buddhism follows idealistic metaphysics. It starts its speculation by taking the existence of the subject alone as the base (as in Western philosophy). It then analyses the existence of the world from the viewpoint of this subject, which is the first order of existence. There are three schools of Mahayana Buddhism, which represent three stages of idealistic logic: *Sautantrika*, *Yogachara*, and *Madhyamika*.

In Sautantrika, students accept the subject (the individual consciousness) first and then analyze the world from this viewpoint. They then go on to accept the existence of the world on the ground of inference, by inferring it from our common sense. Both the subject and the world, as in Hinayana Buddhism, exist in themselves, and there is no absolute beyond them. Sautantrika Buddhism is usually classified under Hinayana, but being the first of the idealistic positions it would be better to class it under Mahayana Buddhism. In Yogachara they are more logical and do not accept the outside world at all, and say the subject (the individual consciousness) is the sole reality, and all else is a dream of the mind. In Yogachara, the mind is the only reality. In Madhyamika (to be differentiated from Mahayana), they follow the strictest logic, and deny the existence of both the object and the subject, and declare *shunya* as the only truth.

A variant of Mahayana Buddhism that developed in China and Japan is Zen Buddhism, which follows Yogachara logic and says that only the mind or consciousness exists, and the pure undifferentiated state of consciousness is the only truth. Zen Buddhism differs from Mahayana Buddhism in that it lays stress mainly on meditation, in which students try to experience this undifferentiated state

> *Looking for the Maker of this tabernacle, I shall have to run through a course of many births, so long as I do not find (Him); and painful is birth again and again. But now, Maker of the tabernacle, thou hast been seen; thou shalt not make up.*
>
> —Dhammapada 153, 154

Hinayana or Theravada Buddhism is considered the original Buddhism, and is truer to Buddha's teachings. In Theravada Buddhism the world is called *samsara*, and it is the main focus of all Buddhist speculation. Buddha taught that the samsara is dukha, or full of suffering, and that this suffering can be got rid of. But if the suffering can be got rid of, there must be nothing permanent in it. Hence the world was said to be relative or a "dependent reality," or *pratitya samutpada*; that is, the world does not have any other support, but instead subsists on itself. One thing supports another, and that in turn supports some other thing, and so on, without any base in absolute reality. For example, death and suffering comes from birth, birth comes from craving, and so on, with none of them having any individual reality.In the famous metaphor of Nagarjuna, the world was described as a circle of light formed by a firebrand that is whirled about. The circle does not really exist and is formed by multiple positions of the firebrand, but when we see it we do not see the individual positions of the firebrand but the circle as a whole. In the same way, the samsara also consists of fragments but we see it as a whole and as a reality.

Because there is no reality beyond it, the world is an illusion—something that exists but has no true reality, like the circle of fire. It has what we might call a "fuzzy" or blurred reality only. This illusion is called *maya* in Buddhism. The duty of humans is to pierce through this veil of maya and recognize that the world is only this pratitya samutpada. The world will not then cease to exist, but once the truth is known, maya will lose its power and we will achieve inner peace and tranquility, or nirvana.

Thus Hinayana or Theravada Buddhism defines a metaphysical position in which Advaitism is rejected, as there is no absolute beyond the world, and at the same time nihilism is rejected, because the world does exist as a self-supporting entity. This concurs well with Buddha's teachings, which say that there is no intrinsic reality to dukha, while also rejecting nihilism. The world, or samsara, existing as a dependant reality, is the only truth.

If there is nothing beyond this world and this world is only a dependant reality, then how does the world sustain itself? Buddhist philosophers explained the existence of the world as a momentary existence. For example, if we take a young man who has changed into an old one, what exactly has happened? At the end of the process, there is an old man and not the young one, and this old man is certainly a different entity from the young one. He is different in his looks, thoughts, voice, and so forth. The Buddhists cannot accept a gradual, continuous change from a young man into an old, because if the change is continuous, then it means something—that is, the man—continuously existed. This would mean eternalism, because we can then say something continues to exist for eternity; even after the man dies, first his body will continue to exist, and then the atoms and the molecules.

Thus the Buddhists explained it by saying that there is continuous replacement of changes—that is, the young man disappears and the old one appears in his stead. But this change is continuous; hence there must be a series of continuous changes. Thus the Buddhists say that at every moment the previous man disappears and a slightly older one appears in his stead. Since this change appears continuous, the change must be taking place at a very fast rate, several times in a moment.

This is rather like a movie reel; we think we see the picture moving, but the pictures actually do not move. Instead it is a series of still pictures that are each slightly different from the previous and, when run quickly together, appear to move. So also in the world, there is no continuous change but rather a series of interrupted small changes, which to us appear as a continuous change. It is not just matter, but our consciousness also, which instead of a continuous state of awareness consists of a series of "still" impressions that, when run together, give the impression of a continuously existing consciousness. Thus in Buddhism, the world is being continuously created and destroyed several times in each moment, and there is nothing that exists in the gaps. Hence there is nothing that connects one moment to the next and therefore no absolute. This is the Buddhist theory of *Ksanabhangavada* or "momentary existence," as it is called. Through this startling explanation, the Buddhists explain the presence of the world without any absolute beyond it.

What is required is to achieve the state of nirvana. Nirvana, again, is not a state of consciousness, as samadhi in Advaita is defined as a state of existence in Brahman. Instead, nirvana is a state of knowledge, a state in which the meditator acquires the firm and unshakeable true knowledge of the world, that it is only dukha and dependant reality and so on. This stage is achieved by following the precepts of the eightfold path, which lead to a moral and peaceful life, along with intense meditation. Once a person has this reality, he will no more be led by desires. He will then live in a state of complete calmness and tranquility from which nothing can shake him.

Buddhism believes in the theory of reincarnation, and thus it is said that those souls that have not achieved this nirvana or knowledge of shunya are reborn again. They must continue to suffer this state of rebirth until they obtain the state of nirvana. Once this knowledge is acquired, a person will not be reborn ever again and will be freed from the cycle of dukha or suffering. This is the end; this is the supreme goal of Buddhism. This is the ideal state and Buddha was born in order to help all to achieve this state.

Buddhism, which at one time was the dominant religion of India, virtually disappeared from India from around the ninth century. Many reasons are given for this mystery, including that it was subsumed by the parent religion and the rise of Bhaktism. But one of the most important reasons undoubtedly is the inherent deficiency in Buddhist logic, which was attacked by Advaitists, most notably Shankara, and eventually led to the conversion of the majority of Buddhist scholars to Advaitism.

It is in fact difficult to accept the very first dictum of Buddhism, that the world is dukha or suffering. The Buddhist view that everything in the world is dukha, that we all have the arrow of sadness in our hearts and need to get rid of this arrow, seems a very depressing view of life. Granted, people are not happy all the time in the world, but it does seem too much for anyone to tell us that our life is one long tale of constant suffering. When there are so many beautiful things in life—love, poetry, music, the wonder of flowers and mountains, the joy of loving someone and of bringing up children—it seems annoying, to say the least, for anyone to say that they are all worthless.

The main aim of Buddhism is to get rid of all our desires—that is, all the hopes and aspirations that pull us along—and to lead a completely detached life. This might seem a great plus to someone to whom all life is negative, but to the vast majority of us, it must look extremely unattractive to forego all that we love and cherish in our lives, even though they may bring us sorrow too sometimes. But it is on this belief that all life is suffering that the whole of the theory and practice of Buddhism is based.

Again, in Buddhism there is nothing that has any reality; everything in the world is unreal. But can the world actually exist as only a dependant reality without any basis to it? The classic answer to the Buddhist theory was given by Gaurapada, the guru of Shankaracharya, who dealt at length with Nagarjuna's Madhyamika analytics. Both Hinayana Buddhism and Advaitism accept that the world is only relatively real, and therefore the arguments and metaphors given by both to support this aspect are the same. But from this initial argument, both arrive at opposite conclusions: one that there is an absolute beyond the world, and the other that there is no absolute.

In response to the metaphor of the circle of fire produced by a brand, which is being whirled about, Gaurapada asked, what about the brand itself? Granted that the circle does not exist and may be considered virtual, yet it still has to have a basis even to have this virtual reality, and that basis is the brand. The circle cannot be produced out of nothingness. So also with this world; if the world itself is only virtual reality, then it has to have a *basis* to exist. Something cannot ever be nothing, so to say; the world and existence have to have a ground to stand on. The world cannot be unreal through and through. One unreal thing cannot go on to support another unreal phenomenon, and so on, like two men lifting each other up into the sky by pulling each other's hair. Buddhism contradicts not only logic but also our common sense, as it is impossible to see how a world that has only relative reality can exist without anything beyond it.

Buddhism is sometimes seen to be very similar to Jainism, as both accept only the world and seek to know it and no other. But ultimately it differs in a fundamental way from Jainism because it denies the reality of the world. To support the theory of unreality of the world and deny any continuity, Buddhists proposed the theory of Ksanabhangavada, but this seems to pose more problems than it solves.

The Buddhist view of existence as Ksanabhangavada is that it is all something that comes from nothing, exists for an infinitesimally small point of time, and relapses into nothing. Nothing has independent existence and all things are related to the existence of something else, which in turn would be dependent on something else, and so on. The Buddhists are forced to say that there is no connection between the moments because that would mean that the world has continuous existence, and hence it would lead to eternalism.

But Advaitists pointed out that such a theory has several deep flaws, besides being contrary to all our intuition. In the first place, if there is indeed no connection between two moments of existence, then how is it that the same order in the world is reproduced each time? There might as easily have been chaos with different worlds and events being produced at each moment. What is there that holds it together? In the same way, because each moment of our consciousness is also momentary, how is it that we have memory? Since each impression is being destroyed at each moment, we should have lost all our previous impressions.

Again, Buddhists are forced to accept that each moment of existence is infinitesimally small, for if the world can be said to exist for even a microsecond of time, then there is no bar to saying that it can exist for a second, and hence eventually to existence. If they accept any length of existence, then that too would lead to eternalism. This then raises many problems, such as how such infinitely small moments could add up to any length of time, whether time exists in the gaps, and so on. These and several other flaws based on similar arguments were pointed out by the opponents of Buddhism.

The Buddhist view that birth or the new origination of things in the world denied nihilism and that death denied absolutism ignored one key fact, that there was neither true origination nor true destruction. When a thing is born or is originated, it does not come out of nothing; it is merely a change in the state of elements that had already existed before, and that are now coming together in a new state. Similarly, death or destruction of a thing does not mean that it has disappeared into nowhere, but simply that its elements are resolved into something else. When a candle burns itself out for example, it does not disappear but is simply changed into different forms of ash, smoke, and energy. Hence there is neither any new creation out of nothing nor any disappearance into nothing, but merely different forms of existence. Birth and death do not mean a new existence or the end of an old one but only a continuity of subsistence. Therefore, in this world there is always a continuity of existence.

The Buddhists chose to answer all such arguments by a stoic silence, merely saying that that is how it is, and it is useless to ask the "how" and "why" of something that *is*. But others continued to ask them, and Buddhists found it difficult to defend their metaphysical theories.

Buddhist beliefs also lead to great problems in our day-to-day life. The Buddhist view is that this world is inherently meaningless, and the only wise thing that anyone could do would be to know it as such. This would make all our science irrelevant. It implies that we are merely being fooled into thinking that the world events are following any order, and we should give up science and go into meditation. So also all the arts, music, and poetry are all irrelevant and worthless in Buddhism

But in Advaita, everything has a basis in reality—that is, Brahman—and everything exists as a differentiation of Brahman. Hence things have a reality, only this reality is relative in contrast to the reality of Brahman, which is absolute. Hence the laws of science work within the relative plane, because the phenomena that they study have a basis in the absolute, and this absolute may be approached by studying the phenomenon, "as by knowing a lump of earth the whole earth may be known." So also the arts, poetry, music, and our daily successes and sorrows all have their own place of relevance. Through each of these, by studying them and understanding them, we can approach the ultimate reality because all have a reflection of the absolute in them. Hence in Hinduism, all things—science, poetry, music, art—have a mystical connotation to them and become vitally important, as they all have the potential of ultimately leading us to the final truth.

Another big disadvantage in Buddhism is the elimination of Bhakti, or love of God, as a practice. There is nothing that is an absolute in this world, nothing that is higher than this world. Hence there is nothing to depend on.

But in Advaita, the absolute is recognized, and hence this absolute can be approached by personalizing it for the purposes of Bhakti. Bhakti appears to be a universal need for humanity, and cultures in all ages and places have gravitated toward it. It appears to fulfill a deep spiritual need for us. Hence Hindus and Advaitists have the joy of Bhakti as their spiritual force. Ultimately, of course, this personalization of the absolute and Bhakti is left behind when the final culmination of samadhi is achieved in Advaitism.

The Buddhist end goal of religion is also different. Buddhists do not seek a higher dimension in life because, unlike in Advaitism, there is no higher state of existence. What Buddhists seek is higher knowledge. The Buddhist mystical experience, which in fact should not be called mystical in the true sense of the word, is the acquisition of this higher knowledge (that the world is only dependant reality, etc.). Once this knowledge is acquired, the aspirant loses all his desires that kept him bound to the world, and then on death, achieves nirvana, the stage of birthlessness.

Once this knowledge becomes fixed, upon subsequent meditation Buddhists discover more and more facets of samsara or the
world. They come to realize its different categories and diversities
as defined by Buddhism; for example, they categorize the mind
into five different states, then further categories are developed for
the sense organs, the different ways objects strike the sense organs,
and so on. All the phenomena of the world are subdivided into
such categories, with subdivisions galore within each category.
Again, many of the categories, such as "will" and "ether," are ill-
defined and intangible. There is literally no end to such categories,
which the aspirant has to know. As the subject's knowledge of the
untrue nature of the world becomes vaster, he becomes freer and
freer from the world.

However, it would seem that such pursuit of knowledge inherently has its defects, because the subjects of knowledge are vast.
Such a continuous acquiring of knowledge would be never-ending
it seems, and as one goes further, more and more objects of knowledge would keep appearing. The Buddhists judge this as going further and further ahead, because the aspirant becomes wiser in his
knowledge that the world is unreal. But it means essentially that
there is no end to the Buddhist inquiry, and the Buddhist monk
would only get saddled with increasing and interminable knowledge of something that is essentially not worth knowing.

In Advaita, once the experience of oneness with Brahman is
acquired, it is the end and there is no need to acquire further knowledge of the relative world. In the Advaitic samadhi, it is not knowledge that is achieved in the final stage, but the *experience* of a
totally new state of existence, a new state of consciousness. The
world becomes clear as an illusion and the Advaitist does not wish
to have any more knowledge of it. In Buddhism the world does

not disappear in nirvana, and instead we only come to have a true knowledge of it.

Hence Buddhist mysticism is not a different "state of existence," but "knowledge." Of course, this knowledge is not the simple intellectual knowledge but a sort of merger into the knowledge, becoming one with it, which is possible through meditation. Hindu Yoga also recognizes such a state of merger with knowledge, which can be brought about in meditation, and it is called *samyama*. However samyama, or the knowledge state, is not considered the end stage of religion as the objects of knowledge are those of the world itself, and not of that which is higher than this world. Instead the Yogi goes further and achieves a stage of merger with that which is higher than any phenomena of this world. This is the end point of Hinduism; the Buddhist goal in this view is considered only a halfway goal.

The other great branch of Buddhism, which developed in answer to the need to define a metaphysical position following Buddha's teachings, is Mahayana or Sanskrit Buddhism. It developed later than the Theravada, and its scriptures were in Sanskrit, whereas in Hinayana they had been in Pali.

Mahayana Buddhism gradually spread into China due to the efforts of Buddhist monks, and there Buddhism virtually took on a life of its own. Mahayana Buddhism is now found mainly in China, Japan, Korea, and the surrounding regions, and the original school, the Theravada, also called the Hinayana, is found mainly in the South Asian countries like Sri Lanka, Myanmar, Thailand, Vietnam, and so forth. In its original land, India, Hinayana Buddhism was supplanted by Mahayana Buddhism, but it also was ultimately subsumed by Hinduism. The most well-known of the Mahayana schools is Zen Buddhism.

Just think of the trees: they let the birds perch and fly, with no intention to call them when they come and no longing for their return when they fly away. If people's hearts can be like the trees, they will not be off the Way.

—Zen Quotes by Langya

Mahayana Buddhism starts from the position of metaphysical idealism. It accepts, before beginning all speculation, the "I," or the individual mind, as the only true entity and analyses the world from this standpoint. There are three schools of Mahayana: Sautantrika, Yogachara, and Madhyamika. Although Sautantrika is usually classified as a Theravada school, if Mahayana includes all the idealistic schools of Buddhism, then Sautantrika should also fall under it.

The Sautantrikas start from the position of idealism and regard the subject, the "I," as alone being real. But when we consider the subject alone, the thinker alone, to be the first point of existence, then we cannot prove the existence of the world independently of the subject. It may be nothing more than a dream. Nevertheless, the Sautantrikas make a doctrinal jump of logic and accept that the world exists, by inferring it from common sense. Thus, whereas Theravada starts from the realistic position that both the subject and the world are equally real, the Sautantrikas start from the idealistic position that only the subject is real and accept the world as only "inferentially" real. Beyond both these existences, like the Theravada, they say there is no absolute and that the world and the subject exist as dependent realities only. The rest of its philosophy is similar to Theravada, and it differs only in its idealistic starting point metaphysically, due to which it considers the world as "inferentially" real. It thus comes the closest to the Theravada philosophy but for its idealistic standpoint.

The Yogachara school follows the logic of the idealistic metaphysical position more strictly. Here, after starting from the point of the subject alone, it is seen that what we know of the world is only what our minds tell us about it, and we cannot know the world apart from the mind. Hence, logically, the world is nothing more than a creation of the mind. So the Yogachara, by following logic strictly, declare that the world is nothing but a dream of the mind. The only truth is the mind alone, pure consciousness. Even other people are, after all, part of the world outside, and each of us only thinks they exist because our mind tells us so. Thus other people are also creations of the mind. So each person could say "The only truth is *my* mind. *I* alone exist, and this whole world is a dream of my mind."

The mind is constantly creating these images of the world—and, hence, is always in a disturbed state. But if it can break through this dream, the mind will retain its original state of tranquility in which it is totally undisturbed and calm—the state of nirvana. This is done by following the Buddhist eightfold path, and this is the goal of Yogachara.

Yogachara philosophy formed the basis of the Zen Buddhism in China and Japan. Yogachara did not specify whether nirvana was a positive state of realization, but Zen philosophers categorically accepted the One-Mind as a positive entity, which was realized in meditation.

The main reason for this Zen trend toward positivism was the experience of the Zen monks in meditation. Zen texts spoke of the realization of the blissfulness of the pure state or "Suchness" of the mind in the state of samadhi. The most common metaphor given for Zen meditation was the metaphor of the sky and clouds, in which the Zen aspirant thinks of himself as the clear sky, bereft of all existence, while the clouds of phenomena drift past. So Zen teachings eventually became more and more concerned with the state of existence experienced in meditation and less concerned with the nature of the world. Thus the focus of spiritual life is quite different from Theravada.

Zen differs fundamentally from Theravada Buddhism not just in philosophy but also in its practice and meditation. Whereas Theravada seeks only for knowledge of the world, in Zen the aspirants try to find the stillness within themselves. Thus Zen, as in Hinduism, aims for an experience of a "state of existence" rather than a "knowledge." Zen meditation developed in various schools, and many different techniques became prevalent. In general, the thrust is to concentrate on the serenity within oneself while the motion of the world flies past. Zen aspirants try to avoid any active engagement with world events and thus try to distance themselves from them, remaining as mere observers. In this way, as they distance themselves more and more from the world, they approach their inner calmness, the core of the mind, which does not move. Finally, when the aspirant is able to totally distance him or herself from the world, they are one with this stillness and are not affected by the world anymore, thus achieving nirvana.

The Zen students who wish to achieve this try to cultivate this detachment throughout their whole lives. A common Zen teaching used to describe their passage through life is, "I eat when I am hungry, I sleep when I am tired." It means that the aspirants live dispassionately; doing merely what is required of them at that particular instant without any thought of either the future or the past. In this way, the detachment pursued in every act of life becomes a reality.

Zen teachings are also less doctrinal and give more independence for the aspirant as each is encouraged to pursue meditation in his or her own way, and meditation is a more personal task in Zen. Zen is also far more pragmatic, and its rules both for its monks and householders are far less strict.

Yogachara and Zen, however, faced some vital problems in their philosophies. For one thing, it is almost impossible to accept the astounding idea suggested by such extreme solipsism. That the world does not exist and is only a dream of my mind is something that flies in the face of all our convictions. The whole outside world in all its physical and social aspects, including science, the arts, and social relationships with other people, along with the sun, moon, and other surroundings, are apparently all only a bad dream that I am having, and I am only dreaming even as I laugh, talk, learn new things, walk about, and so forth. Theories like the evolutionary theory, which would contradict such idealism because it says that the mind is evolved from pre-existing matter, would be rejected as another bad dream, along with all other physical sciences, history, logic, and more.

In fact, Zen takes its disregard for logic to extreme lengths. Because things like logic are part of the dream and keep us tied into the dream by making us believe that the world is real, Zen tries to break the cycle of logic. One such way are the Zen riddles called *koans*, which are deliberately irrational. For example, one famous koan goes this way: a monk asked Chao-Chow, "All things return to oneness. Whither does oneness return?" Chao-Chou replied: "When I was staying at Chin Chou, I made a robe of cloth weighing seven pounds." A completely irrational answer is given to the question in the hope that the questioner will realize instantly the uselessness of logic and achieve the pure state.

Another similar technique is that, as the monks are meditating quietly, a teacher goes around the room and gives them a big whack with a stick, so that in the moment of startlement, the student might "break out" of his dream, so to say. A disinterested observer cannot be blamed for asking whether there is really something going on or if it is just an instance of the "emperor's new clothes," with people getting themselves fooled into taking seriously something that would set a child laughing.

In their metaphysics, Zen and Yogachara contradict Buddha's original teachings. He expressly forbade all forms of absolute existence, which would survive for eternity, but these two schools described an eternal and absolute consciousness.

Zen also suffers from other defects of Buddhist philosophy that it has in common with Theravada Buddhism, such as the transitory nature of life, the pessimism regarding life that lies at the heart of its teaching, that all life is dukha, the lack of Bhakti in Buddhism, and more. Regarding the various questions as to whether is there a meaning to life, whether love, poetry, and music have any value, and whether science is valid, all these questions would elicit a "yes" from Advaita, whereas Zen, along with Theravada and Mahayana Buddhism, would say a firm "no." Because Zen defines the world as dream-like, all things connected with the world are said to take one away from the truth. But this attempt to deprive life of all meaning is not, perhaps, the great teaching that most of us are looking for.

The logical endpoint of the metaphysical idealism of Mahayana is the nihilism of the school of Madhyamika. Nihilism, a denial of existence, may be said to be of many types: spiritual or moral nihilism, which would deny any moral or spiritual values; political nihilism, which would negate all political systems; social nihilism, which would deny the importance of social structures; and so on. In the context of metaphysics, metaphysical nihilism would deny the existence of this world.

Spiritual or moral nihilism says that nothing in the world has any *value*; the world is temporary and so are all our lives, and hence any attempt to find a higher goal in life by following an ethical code or a set of religious teachings is a vain attempt. Materialists are such nihilists, and in India the *Charvakas* were the most influential of such schools.

If there is no higher truth beyond the world, if the world is all there is, then all spiritual concepts are also only a part of the world and are hence artificial concepts. They do not rest on any ultimate truth, and are merely man-made teachings, which may or may not be accepted. The Buddhists and the Jains were most susceptible to the Charvaka's logic, because they taught that the world was all the reality and there was no higher truth beyond the world. They preached that nirvana did not lead one to a higher state; it merely signified an escape from what was considered a negative state into a state of nothingness, or from minus to zero, so to speak. The Charvakas contended that if there was no higher truth or higher experience, then leading a hedonistic life and trying to get the maximum out of this life itself was just as tenable as trying to know it or escape from it. Modern scientific agnosticism is also as susceptible to Chavaka logic.

The famous Charvaka saying was, "eat *ghee*, even if you have to borrow," meaning that life should be enjoyed to the fullest. The Charvakas attacked not only the metaphysical positions but also, more specifically, the moral, ethical, and religious values of different belief systems, exposing the vulnerability behind their logic. This led both the Buddhists and Jains to launch a vitriolic attack against such nihilism, which was presumably returned as strongly. Little of the Charvaka teachings survive today, and we come to know of them mainly from the intense criticism they were subjected to in Buddhist and Jain literature.

Advaitism escapes from such moral nihilism because it asserts the existence of a higher truth to the world, the absolute. This absolute lies behind everything, and hence the world is not a meaningless entity but one that is based on solid ground. Moreover, all things—poetry, science, arts, human relationships, and so on—become things of value because they all are ultimately based on this absolute and can lead us to it.

The most radical position among all metaphysical systems is that of the radical Buddhist nihilists, the Madhyamikas, who deny the existence of not just the external world but of the subject as well. This is the most logical of all the schools that start from the position of metaphysical idealism, that the subject by itself is the first existence, and it is they alone who follow the argument to its cold, stark end. They argue that if the world is only a dream, then the "flashes" of memories, sensations, and so forth are also not real, as they are only delusions. If the dream world is unreal, it is impossible to show that the waking world, its equivalent, is real; if the waking world also is unreal, then the subject, whose existence is defined by this waking world, must also be unreal. Because consciousness consists only of these "flashes" of memories, sensations, and so on of the waking world, the subject too is a mere delusion if these flashes are unreal. True religion, therefore, consists of overcoming this delusion, thus resulting in a complete nullification of all existence.

This void is called shunya among the Madhyamikas. Shunya here does not mean a *state* of nothingness or emptiness; rather, it is something that does not exist. To use an awkward word, it is an "unfindable." It is not that there is a higher truth, which is shunya or emptiness; it is that there is no higher truth beyond this world. Shunya does not describe anything but is merely a word signifying absence. It is akin, as the Upanishads describe it, to the "children of a barren woman" or the "horns of a hare," something that by definition does not exist. This doctrine, that all existence is ultimately shunya, is the main doctrine of the Madhyamikas.

The Madhyamikas were able to establish a formidable philosophical position, which was difficult to contradict if one followed their doctrines. Many questions can be raised against such nihilism—such as how we are all having the same dream, who is dreaming, where did the dreams begin and how—but all these arise only later. Once we start from the position of "I"-ism, or metaphysical idealism, it becomes impossible to escape from the logic of absolute nihilism, and we are forced to accept its conclusions even if many questions remain unanswered. Absolute nihilism is the only logical end point of metaphysical idealism, and the unrelenting logic of the Madhyamikas made them end up with this position. Madhyamikas do not try to defend their position so much as attack all other positions and disprove any attempts to prove existence, which is impossible in metaphysical idealism.

Ultimately nihilistic Buddhism, as with all nihilism, would always remain on the fringes of spiritual thought because of the sheer unreasonableness of its teachings. It goes against all our instincts to accept that things around us do not exist. It robs any meaning from life, and makes us look foolish. No force of logic could make us swallow this bitter pill. But the sheer logic of their arguments, which make their conclusions inescapable once we start from the position of metaphysical idealism, made nihilistic Buddhism a powerful philosophy; it survived because it was simply impossible to kill it off.

The Upanishads, like Theravada Buddhism, avoids nihilism because it starts from metaphysical realism and does not accept the starting point of metaphysical idealism, the prior existence of the "I" alone. Instead it accepts the simultaneous existence of the trio of knower, knowledge, and the thing that is known, and analyses the world from this viewpoint. Hence we arrive at a logical and harmonious understanding of the world.

It must be realized that there is a great deal of controversy regarding the actual teachings of these Buddhist schools. The texts are very large in number and their meanings are ambiguous and contradictory, so that virtually any sort of meaning can be twisted out from them. Various commentators interpreted them in their own ways, to try to make them more "satisfactory." Perhaps the very fact that there are so many controversies and no agreement regarding the actual teaching of any of the Buddhists schools shows up the weakness in their logic, and gives a hint as to why Buddhism eventually could not stand up against Hindu logic and was absorbed into Hinduism.

Thus of all the various positions arrived at in various schools of thought, Advaitism appears as the most balanced. It does not call for any doctrinal beliefs but is a position that can be arrived at by simple logical arguments. At the same time, it endows everything in our lives with a deeper meaning, and makes them vitally important in our struggle for spiritual growth. Advaitism provides the theoretical basis for the final experience of Hinduism, samadhi, in which we unite with the great truth that lies behind us. At the same time, all forms of philosophical arguments have their own roles to play in this tapestry of human thought. A knowledge of all these undoubtedly helps us in our efforts for understanding the mystery of our existence.

Advaita and Modern Knowledge

*Knowledge and ignorance are different. Only that which is
done with knowledge, faith and meditation, that alone becomes
more powerful. This truly is the proximate exposition of this
very letter Om.*

—Chandogya Upanishad I.i.10

The scientific analysis of the world, depending not just on
logical analysis but on observation and experiments, has
thrown up a whole new dimension of our existence. The
old religious and metaphysical theories have been thrown into ferment, and only the more rigorous ones can survive now. In fact, the
further development of science is likely to challenge most other
metaphysical theories. Among the different metaphysical positions, only one can be true, and ultimately we will be led into
accepting the position that is in conformity with both logic and
scientific knowledge.

The whole gamut of philosophy has been well-covered through
the ages, and there seems hardly any gap in theory. The result is a
confusing mass, with different theories often being united at one
point and virulently opposed at some other point. It is, in fact,
often difficult to differentiate one theory from the other, or to
remember all the subtle details in them.

Faced with the mass of metaphysical theories, we may ask, why should we not believe our initial view of the world as really existing, and be satisfied with it? Why should we ask questions like whether the world is real or not? A candle exists, burns, and dissipates as smoke and ash. Granted that the candle is impermanent, but why should we consider its reality or unreality? It is certainly real as long as it exists, and even after it dissipates, the smoke and ash are real as long as *they* exist. It is true that we do not know everything about the world; when we see a flower, for example, we cannot know all the details, and we merely form a partial impression of it. Similarly, all other people form a partial impression of it and do not know it in totality, and nor do all the impressions match, because it varies with the person who is observing it. Granted that we all have relative *knowledge* only of the flower, but it does not mean that the flower itself has only relative *reality*. It is only because we do not have perfect faculties that we do not see the flower in its full reality, but it can still have one. Although our knowledge of the world is partial, it is still a world that is real in itself and there is no reason to doubt it or to look for something beyond it.

This is the commonsense view, and it is the view of modern pantheism, or scientific pantheism, which gained wide currency in the nineteenth century following the new advancements in science. This is in fact a qualified monism position, and is virtually identical with Jainism. Most other religions, including Taoism and Tantricism, can also be considered to be qualified monistic views. They are of course all different in some subtle ways, but the common belief that ties them is that this world is real, all things in the world are a part of a larger reality, and this reality as a whole is eternal, infinite, and many-sided, and is the goal of our spiritual quest. There is no higher reality apart from this universe. This infinite reality of the universe has no will and is not a creator. It simply exists, and our known world is a part of this existence.

Scientific pantheism has no place for souls or any other such enigmatic phenomena. There is some difference, though, in the understanding of different pantheist schools, and some see a primal difference between mind and matter. Some schools again consider matter as the primary element, and make the mind only a function of matter, while some consider mind to be the primary element and make matter a function of it.

Pantheism was given a firm base by the new scientific discoveries of the nineteenth century, and it became a kind of new, scientific religion. The physics of Newton and other discoveries of that period depicted a grand harmonic universe in which everything had its own place and importance. Other theories, such as the theory of evolution, again led to a mechanistic interpretation of life and our role in the world. All this leads to the conception that the universe is the ultimate reality and there is nothing above the universe. The universe itself then becomes the object of worship. The spiritual quest in pantheism is to become one with the beauty and majesty of the universe. The goal is to seek this beauty everywhere in nature and to cultivate a deep sense of reverence, and even a mystical experience, when in contact with this beauty.

However, nature worship by itself cannot be the end of our spiritual quest. It is not difficult to see the deep sense of reverence that a scene from nature might evoke, but to take this as the goal of religion seems to be going too far. Nature is hardly all beauty and kindness, nor does it always evoke an "overwhelming sense of power and beauty." Such a religion does not take us very far beyond an idealistic worship of beauty. It cannot give us any of the things such as spiritual strength and a higher ideal that we seek from a religion.

Also on the practical side is the actual worshipping of nature. The wonders of nature are grand indeed, but it is rather naïve to see only the grandness and not the wantonness of nature. A rainbow might seem very grand and beautiful, but when once we see it as nothing more than the diffraction of sunlight by raindrops, it is difficult to get spiritual exaltation from it. So also we would scarcely feel the beauty of nature in the forests if we think of the cruelty of animals and insects to each other.

The pantheistic position, along with all other qualified monistic positions, came to be totally contradicted by modern science. When we examine the world logically, we find the world cannot be explained as being complete in itself; instead we arrive at a theory of some common basis for all phenomena in this world. This leads on logically to the Advaitic view of an absolute reality beyond all phenomena. This was the view arrived at by many Jain scholars, so that some Jain texts are virtually identical with the Advaitic view. In science, also, relativity suggests that there is no absolute time or space, and also that all qualities of a body, such as m/ass, length, and speed, are relative. Quantum physics again has showed us that all things (mass, energy, etc.) are interrelated, and by themselves do not have any absolute existence. All this suggests logically that there is some *constant*, which connects everything together. Hence it would not be enough to know this world alone, which has a nebulous reality, but rather we should try to know this basis *beyond* the world. Hence, with the progress of science, pantheism lost its initial appeal for the rational mind.

The development of science contradicted much of religious thought. But even before this attack, there have always been views that have stood against religion. Nihilism, of course, is one important such view. Besides this, other views that deny religion include agnosticism and atheism.

Agnosticism is the position that it is useless to try and seek anything that is beyond nature, or to seek a higher truth beyond nature, because humans are incapable of knowing anything beyond nature. Buddha's agnosticism is also sometimes interpreted in this way, that he meant to say that it is impossible to know if there is something beyond nature (more commonly, he is interpreted as saying that there was no need to even attempt to find out whether there is something, because it would not be of any practical help).

All our senses, our faculties of knowledge, and therefore our knowledge itself, have evolved to make sense of the niche that we survive in. Thus our minds will never be able to grasp something that is beyond this niche—that is, beyond the natural world. For example, we have developed a concept of time that is most suitable for our survival. All our knowledge and thinking is tied up inextricably with this concept of time, and we can never understand a concept that is timeless or unrelated to time. It is likewise so with our other concepts, such as space. Hence agnostics do not try for knowledge of these things, and instead try to find out about the natural world through scientific inquiry.

But agnosticism does not seem a satisfying position. In the first place, human nature itself is such that, as soon as a question is said to be unanswerable, we are torn by the desire to find that answer. Our history has been shaped by our passion for mystery and adventure and the desire of the mind to always stretch further and push at the boundaries that limit it. It is simply not possible for us to be satisfied with a position where we decide not to enquire further into the questions that most confound us. A closer look at the world around us shows that our initial view is not correct, and we then feel forced to enquire what the correct view is. Only someone who has lost this sense of the mystique and wonder at the universe, which surrounds us, could simply will himself or herself into not looking deeper into it.

Again, although it is true that we can understand only the concepts familiar with our senses, it is not that we cannot even conceive of things beyond senses. In fact practically all of modern physics describes a world far beyond our senses. This knowledge has been acquired through the scientific method of observation and inference, and cannot be said to be invalid or inadequate. The scales of magnitude and time described both in quantum physics and in astronomical science are way beyond our sense appreciation, yet such concepts are regularly discussed and understood throughout the world. Many other concepts of science are not understood by our sense experience, yet this does not make them fallacious in any way.

Similarly, philosophers, through rigid application of logic and inference, can arrive at conceptions of things beyond the senses. In this way, although it is difficult to explain the absolute in common language, understanding a concept of absolute existence is not beyond the capacities of the human mind. Indeed, if we can understand concepts like those discussed in present-day quantum physics, then having a concept of an absolute should not be difficult at all!

Agnosticism basically arose against doctrinal concepts like a willed God and souls, which were, by definition, beyond human understanding. But the concepts of religions such as Advaitism and Buddhism are not such intangible things, which depend only on doctrines and do not allow a logical examination. The Advaitic

Brahman is something that is the ground of all matter, and hence any inquiry into matter will inevitably lead to an inquiry into Brahman. Brahman is not something that is disconnected from matter, and the world is not disconnected from Brahman.

Hence even a scientific inquiry into the material world will have to contend as to whether it accepts the Advaitic idea of a ground beyond all matter or the Buddhist idea of no ground. In our journey into metaphysics we inevitably have to decide whether the absolute exists or not, even when we call it indescribable. To say at this stage that we cannot enquire further because we will not ever know for sure is to pre-answer the question without really trying. Such a position can only be maintained by a sort of doctrinal agnosticism, as opposed to a modern scientific attitude.

Another position that is against religion is atheism. Atheism is the theory that says there is no God. Atheism denies the concept of God that is conventionally described in popular religions. This is a god with a will, a personal god, who is influenced by and guards over us, and also at one time or the other has had contact with the human race, usually through a special messenger or by taking birth directly. It is easy to see how such fairytales will not easily convince a person of reason. Any number of arguments can be raised against such gods, as they defy all logic and rationality.

But not all gods are defined as such. The metaphysical positions of Buddhism, Advaitism and also such religions as pantheism and Jainism, do not describe such a God. In fact, such religions may well be considered to be atheistic themselves, and were even condemned as such by others. Atheism is valid only against a concept of a personal God, and becomes irrelevant against more logical positions.

The infinite is where one does not see anything else, does not
hear anything else and does not understand anything else.
Hence the finite is where one sees something else, hears
something else, and understands something else.

—Chandogya Upanishad VII.xxiv.1

Again, we might ask, what does it matter what metaphysical position we accept? What does it matter whether we believe there is an absolute or not, whether we believe there is a willed god or not?

The answer is that these metaphysical differences are vital in our spiritual quest, and also impact on our practical life in many subtle ways. To a dualist, the world is created by a willed god, and he or she strives for this god, and the world is useful only as an indicator of the god's greatness. To the qualified monists, the world *is* the god, and they worship this world itself as a part of the larger reality.

To the Advaitists, the absolute that lies beyond this world is the goal, and this absolute is not a personal god, so their methods of worship are more intellectual. To the Buddhist, the world is a falsity, and by knowing this in totality, we can achieve inner calm and tranquility. To those who consider themselves atheists or agnostics, there is no spiritual quest whatsoever and the world is seen only on a day-to-day basis.

The difference in metaphysical positions translates into different ways of looking at the world, and hence shapes our values and ideals. It is ingrained into our psyche that we seek for higher things, whether we do it through science and logic or through religion. We always seek that which is true. Hence in our search for an ideal metaphysical position also, we must strive for that which is supported by logic, rationality, and scientific inquiry. It is only when our ideal is not contradicted by other truths that we can derive not just spiritual strength, but also an intellectual basis for religion.

Modern scientific discoveries have been a sort of victory for Advaitism and Buddhism. The Advaitists, as well as the Buddhists, described the world as having only an ill-defined, blurred reality. Ideas like absolute time, absolute space, determinative laws of cause and effect, change, and so forth were all seen to be logically inconsistent. Hence such ideas could not be true. But if they were false, then the true reality of the world was one where such ideas did not apply. Thus the world did not have such things as absolute time, space, and determinative laws of cause and effect, and hence was an ill-defined world. This was how the ancient seers of the Upanishads had decrypted the world in the meditative insights, and hence it was also supported by knowledge gathered in meditation, which in Hinduism is of supreme importance.

This idea, that the world is in reality an ill-defined, nebulous world, was a cornerstone of Advaitism and Buddhism, and had always attracted much criticism from other philosophies. It was considered a play of words, or an impractical and improvable thesis. Early Western philosophers were quick to see in this a typical Indian attitude of navel gazing and slothfulness. The world around us seems "solid" and real, and we find it almost impossible to believe that it is some kind of a blurred, amorphous shadow only.

But now modern scientific discoveries have also uncovered just such a view of the world. It is interesting that, while no amount of logic or reason can convince opposing philosophers, very few would doubt an observation by a scientist. With all the strength of arguments at its command, the view of the unreality of the world remained at best a fringe view for thousands of years, but within a few years of scientists also declaring the same, the idea has come to be widely accepted.

The first suggestion that our ideas of "classical" reality described by Newton and others, in which a solidly real world existed in an absolute time and space, were wrong was given by the theory of relativity. Einstein showed that there was in fact no absolute time and space, and so a vital part of our belief in traditional dualistic and qualified monistic metaphysics fell through. No object in the universe has absolute mass, length, breadth, or speed.

Whenever we describe an object as having a certain mass or a certain length, that mass or length is true only for that observation. It is not universally true. Another observation would give a different mass and length, and yet both these different figures for mass or length would be equally true; we cannot consider either of them as being absolutely true and the other as a deceptive figure. The body thus does not have any absolute mass or an absolute length; all figures for its mass or length are only relatively true. This also applies to its breadth, speed, and so on. Similarly, the laws of physics such as Newton's laws of motion are also not absolute and do not work in every sphere. They are true only in certain circumstances (e.g., when the speed of the bodies is much less than light in Newton's laws)

Next, quantum physics showed that not just time and space, but matter and energy themselves were also blurred and did not have absolute realities. It showed that the quantum particles did not have a well-defined reality; particles were shown to have properties of both matter and energy *at the same time*, which is mutually contradictory. A particle is not considered to have fixed existence at any point of space and time, but rather has a fuzzy existence. The Heisenberg's Uncertainty Principle showed that when we measure the speed of a particle, we cannot know its position, and when we measure the position, we cannot know the speed.

This is not just because our instruments are clumsy and we cannot measure without knocking or disturbing the particles. In fact, the uncertainty holds even for theoretical and mathematical calculations. This is because the particle by itself does not have an absolute form; it depends on how the reaction is analyzed. We cannot pinpoint a point of space or time where a particle exists; we can only give a statistical account of the probability of its existence at a certain point.

For example, in an orbit of an electron around a nucleus, the electron is not considered to be a definite particle whizzing around the nucleus but rather an amorphous, diffuse existence that exists simultaneously at all points of the orbit, different areas having different probabilities of its existence. Because of the "fuzziness" of these particles, the laws deducing their interactions are also fuzzy. We can never pinpoint the exact result of any interaction; we can only give a range of results with different probabilities, any of which may occur without there being any apparent predilection for a particular outcome. Experiments showed that the laws of mechanics were by nature random in the quantum world, and hence there was no determinative law of cause and effect. Thus quantum physics has also shown that all existence has an ill-defined, approximate reality, which does not have any absolute to it.

Such a concept at the same time effectively rules out qualified monism, like pantheism and Jainism, where the world is considered to have a dynamic, harmonious *reality* in space and time. Quantum physics describes one aspect of the universe, the tiniest parts, and says it does not have absolute reality. Special relativity examines another part, the world of very fast movement, and says the world is not absolutely real in that aspect also.

Advaita (and Buddhism) goes much further than this. Advaita predicts that, similarly, the world in every aspect will turn out to have only a hazy and non-absolute reality. The world that we see around us, although appearing at first as a harmonious reality, is in actual fact a non-absolute, non-defined reality only, and as science explores further and further into the world, it will find this determinism—this reality—dissolving into unreality everywhere. This is what Advaita would predict for the development of science.

The descriptions of reality in quantum physics and in Advaitism and Buddhism are startlingly similar. The basic idea of quantum physics is that classical ideas such as matter and energy, which we use normally to describe the world around us, are inappropriate to describe the world in actuality, and that the world cannot be classified by these ideas. The same philosophy is also ascribed to in both Advaitism and Buddhism. In the Upanishads, the true reality, the absolute in this case, is described as "not this, not this." The idea here is that no classical idea is sufficient or adequate to describe the reality. The Buddha describes the reality of the world in this way: "Of this world, it cannot be said either that it 'exists,' 'not exists,' 'both exists and not exists' and 'neither exists nor not exists.'" This conveys in a figurative sense virtually the same sense of reality that quantum physicists seek to communicate. The sutras of these ancient religions and the explanations of modern sciences have now come a full circle. Whereas they were once considered opposed to each other, new synergies are being discovered between science and these ancient religions.

In our everyday view of the world, we do not see the world as an ill-defined reality. We see it as an orderly, defined reality. But in Advaita, there *is no such determinative reality* anywhere. There is no limiting line where an indeterminate, quantum world changes into an orderly classical world, it is all a turbulent fuzzy world. The same indeterminate, ill-defined reality without any laws such as cause and effect is as true for the macroscopic world as it is for the subatomic. This classical reality that we see and experience around us is a delusion. Now, where does this delusion come from? Why does the world not appear to us as it really is, as an ill-defined shadow, and instead seems like an orderly, harmonious reality?

Advaita says that our existence itself determines that that sphere of existence will be coherent for us. If we had existed in a much smaller world, as subatomic particles, for example, then *that* world would have seemed real and orderly for us, or if we had existed in a sphere with very high gravity for instance, or at speeds near that of light, that world then would have seemed coherent for us. The sphere of our existence determines our interaction with the world around us, and ensures that it seems to be orderly and coherent. Our existence, our consciousness, has evolved in a certain sphere, and within it, it has had to learn to make sense. So our consciousness is such that it sees the world around us as coherent. Consciousness and the sense of coherence or harmony of the world have risen simultaneously; they could not have done so otherwise.

It is the nature of the universe that for everything that exists, the world "around" it will appear to be orderly and harmonious. In the world of Hiranyagarbha, the world of gods, the world of humans appears discordant and chaotic, while the heavens appear to be harmonious to a much greater extent. It is only when the plane of the absolute is reached that we see that everything that exists is in fact disharmonious, and only the absolute is real.

This delusion, where we see the unreal world as real, is called *avidya* in Advaita. The fact that the world exists in such a fuzzy state is called *maya*; that is, when we say "This world is maya," we mean that the world exists in this unreal state. In Advaitism, maya stands for the fact that the world exists as an ill-defined reality with the absolute at the base. In Buddhism it signifies the ill-defined reality alone.

> *O good-looking one, by what logic can existence verily come out of non-existence? But surely, O good looking one, in the beginning all this was Existence, One only, without a second.*
> —Chandogya Upanishad VI.ii.2

After thus describing a world that is now found to be very much in agreement with modern science, Advaita then goes further than modern science and asks the final question: can such an ill-defined, amorphous world subsist in itself? In Advaitism it cannot, and there is an absolute reality beyond this on which all this rests. In (Theravada) Buddhism, however, the world can and does subsist in itself, even though it is ill-defined. Science in general has not yet arrived at the question of whether there is an absolute reality or not and the question remains undefined.

This is the age-old question between Advaitism and Buddhism. Both have defined an ill-defined, indeterminate state as the reality of the world. But Advaita asks how such a world can hold together, and says this is possible only because of the absolute field beyond it all. This field "holds" together everything, as it were, and prevents things from "straying," so that the world remains in this indeterminate state without collapsing into complete disorder. The basic difference between Advaita and Buddhism is that in Buddhism, the changing phenomenal world is the basic structure, whereas in Advaita, there is something beyond, and this is the absolute.

Buddhists propose a world that exists in itself, even though its constituents are unreal and contradictory. There is no higher reality; this world has what is called *dependent reality*. Thus even if a particular process has only a relative reality and subsists between reality and unreality, it changes into another, which is again unreal, and so on, forming a self-illusory world that subsists in itself. There is no absolute existence in the world; the objects depend for their reality not on any fundamental reality but on each other.

In Advaita on the other hand, an illusion cannot sustain another illusion. If this world is illusory, then there must be something true beyond it, if the world is relative, there must be an absolute beyond it. Advaita asks, how things, which are by themselves unreal, can give support to any other thing. There must be a base reality somewhere for all this world to exist. The world is not completely understandable in itself. Even the fire circle needs the firebrand, the mirage needs the oasis, the snake needs the rope. Hence in Advaita, the world has an absolute beyond it.

Again, this base reality in Advaita cannot be *in* the world. The world itself is considered to be illusory and without any absolute in it. This base must be *beyond* the world; it must be beyond space, time, and causation, and hence is an absolute reality. Such an absolute reality, which is the basis of the world, is the Brahman.

Advaita would not agree with a qualified monistic view of physics in trying to find a basic reality in the individual building blocks. Newton, and even Einstein when he tried to contradict quantum physics, tried to find a reality in things such as electrons and nuclei. But in Advaita whatever exists individually cannot have a true reality. Such reality for Advaitism could exist only in the basic field, which is universal and absolute and is not separated into blocks.

Of course, "Brahman is beyond the world" does not mean that it is separate from the world, that it is a fundamentally different reality from the world. Brahman is interred into every part of the world; everything that exists in the world is but an aspect of the absolute which lies beyond space, time and causation. All things are but a limited aspect of this absolute. By saying that "it is beyond the world," the Advaitists only mean that the absolute is not accessible to our senses or to our conceptions, because we can only experience and describe that which is relative and limited. But everything, including space and time, is only an outgrowth, as it were, on this reality, like the snow on the mountain peak. It is the source of everything.

If such a reality is not assumed, then the world fails to satisfy us logically. In relativity the Advaitist asks whether, if all time, space, and causation is relative, then would this relative world have been able to sustain itself? There must be something beyond all space and time, in which these qualities are embedded. Because time and space are relative for the entire universe, there must be something beyond the universe itself that is free from time, space, and causation.

Similarly, in quantum physics, Advaitists ask, if each individual particle does not have any well-defined existence, then how can the sum of all this lead eventually to existence? The world cannot be said to be nonexistent either. There must be something that has true existence. Because this true existence is not seen in anything in the world itself, this something must be beyond the world, and from which all others are derived in an ill-defined way, and which gives everything its basis. Because nothing—objects, events, even the law of cause and effect—is absolutely true in itself, all such relative things cannot exist in themselves and must depend on something else, something absolute which is not affected by things such as space and time.

The same point also arises when we consider whether things have a common basis or not. A very important discovery of quantum physics is that matter and energy are interchangeable; matter can be transformed into energy and vice-versa. This was one of the most important principles of physics stated by Einstein in his formula $E=MC^2$. This finding has a profound effect in supporting the Advaitic view of the world. In the Newtonian view, the world was composed of matter and energy, two separate and individually existing entities, so there was no question of some common entity beyond them both. But in quantum physics, the world is ultimately seen not to be composed of different entities but the same spectrum of existence. Both matter and energy are found to be interchangeable, and this implies there must be an ultimate commonality somewhere, something that is common to both matter and energy. It is only if there is something that is common beyond these two (apparently so different) entities that they can interchange into each other. Thus modern physics is in harmony with the Advaitic view of the world. Again, because the universe is fuzzy and ill-defined, this ultimate commonality cannot be present in the universe itself—that is, in either matter or energy. It must be something that is not affected by the universe, something that is beyond the universe. Hence, we arrive at the Advaitic view of the Brahman.

Similarly, when we consider the change of one thing to another, we must ask whether this change is a continuous, smooth change or not. If there is continuity in the world, then there must be a continuous existence somewhere. But because all changes are themselves found to be ill-defined and nebulous, this continuity must be something beyond it, and of which all phenomena and their changes are only manifestations. Continuity of existence is an implied fact of quantum physics, because energy can be considered to be a form of matter and vice versa, and even "empty" space has energy fields. Besides, there is no such thing as a blank space in modern science; space too has such things as curvature that affect matter and energy, and hence ultimately there must be a connection between "blank" space-time and matter-energy.

Thus this continuous existence itself must be beyond change—must be beyond time, space, and causation—for it to support all changes and phenomena. Hence, saying there is continuity or a commonality in the world implies an absolute existence. To avoid this, the Buddhists were constrained to say the world was a discontinuous existence, with their theory of *kshanavrata*, or momentary existence.

Another question is why there is order in the world. If there is nothing in common, then it becomes difficult to see why things are related only in certain ways with other things and not in other, infinite numbers of ways. That is, it is difficult to see how things behave with each other in orderly ways and not in a chaotic fashion. If there was no intrinsic commonality, then there should have been chaos. This is the Advaitic position, and hence they say that the presence of the absolute as the commonality is what makes things behave in an orderly way. As stated in the Katha Upanishad, "For fear of Him fire burns, from fear shines the sun."

Because all things are derived from the same base, they behave in a specific way to each other and hence the universe can be described mathematically.

But because the world is not "well-formed" and is only an approximate reality, the order is not completely determinate; instead, it is based in many fundamental ways on randomness. Hence there is not complete orderly existence in the world but a great deal of indeterminacy. The world exists in this way, between order and indeterminacy, and this is maya.

So logically the conclusions of modern physics, both in relativity and quantum physics, seem to indicate the necessity of an absolute beyond this world, on which this world rests. But experimentally this question is still unresolved. Some theories, such as action-at-a-distance, appear to support such an absolute, while others, such as matrix theory, seem to support the Buddhist view. Science may be said to be noncommittal on this issue, being concerned primarily with finding out the nature of the world, rather than postulating what lies beyond it.

But we can certainly hope that this great dispute will be resolved one day. Already science has shown us the truth or untruth of a great number of religious beliefs. The dispute between the absolute of Advaitism and the "no absolute" of Buddhism lends itself to scientific inquiry, and it seems almost certain that our doubts will be cleared up sooner or later. The Advaitic Brahman is something that is the ground of all matter, and hence any inquiry into matter will inevitably lead to an inquiry into Brahman. Brahman is not something that is disconnected from matter, and the world is not disconnected from Brahman. Hence even a scientific inquiry into the material world will have to contend with whether it accepts the Advaitic idea of a ground beyond all matter or the Buddhist idea of no ground. Just as today we see many religions being disproved by science, future generations will no doubt see either Advaitism or Buddhism disproved, and this will further clear up our search for the ultimate truth.

Of course, according to Advaita, if such an absolute existence is proved, we will still not be able to access it through our material instruments. But perhaps its existence will be indicated in other ways.

The absolute of the Advaita can be described in terms of physics as an absolute field. Most scientists would have no problem with accepting such an absolute field; in fact many would accept it without thinking about it as a religious belief. But Advaita becomes a religion because it says that this absolute forms the basis of our consciousness as well, and, more importantly, that union with this absolute can be achieved in a mystical experience.

> *What was the place whereon he took his station? What was it*
> *that supported him?*
> *He who hath eyes mouth arms and feet on all sides,*
> *He, the Sole God, producing earth and heaven, weldeth them,*
> *with his arms as wings.*
> *What was the tree, what wood in sooth did it produce, from*
> *which they fashioned out the earth and heaven?*
>
> —Rig Veda 10.81

The origin of the universe is another important question that needs to be resolved. In Advaita, the origin and dissolution of the universe is said to happen as a cycle, during a "day" of Brahman, the universe goes through its cycle of creation and dissolution, and following each day there is a "night" of Brahman, when everything remains in an un-manifested state. During the cycle of manifestation, the universe first goes through *nivritti*, or creation, which is compared to an enlarging circle, like the enlarging circle of ripples in a pond. This is completely analogous to the "big bang" theory of the origin of the universe. Then it goes through *pravritti*, which is the same circle closing in. The universe then dissolves completely and Brahman remains in a state of un-manifestation for an equal length of time, after which the cycle begins again.

Modern science also says the same thing; only it does not support this repeated and endless cycle of creation and resolution. But the very fact that the cycle has occurred once indicates that it occurs repeatedly in a circle. Scientists studying the big bang are always trying to determine the first moment of creation, but there cannot be any such moment. Before the first beginning of the big bang, when there was the first step of manifestation, there must have been a moment of disequilibrium that gave rise to creation. If there was no disequilibrium in the system, then it would not have been disturbed at all and there would have been no beginning of the universe. Again, before this first moment of disequilibrium, there must have been another moment of disequilibrium or the first moment could not have begun anew in a stable system. Arguing in this way, we can show that there must have always been a continuous cycle of creation and resolution.

The next question is why this occurs. Why should the universe go through this cycle at all? Here the Advaitists show their supreme naturalism, because in Advaita the cycle is not a willed or directed cycle but occurs naturally. The Brahman of Advaita is not a willed god, and it does not direct this cycle. The Brahman is not affected by these cycles as there is no real change in it, and the manifested universe does not have an absolute reality. It only shows some inconstant properties due to actions of the *upadhis*. During the cycle of un-manifestation, the upadhis do not disappear, because otherwise the creation would not have appeared again. Instead the upadhis remain in a dormant state, and begin creation again at the time of manifestation.

Advaita proposes a most scientific understanding of the universe in that maya, or the nature of the world as it exists, is not ascribed to a supernatural cause. There is no higher power or intelligence that has made the world in this way. The universe evolving in this way is said to be a part of the natural cycle of Brahman; Brahman simply goes through this cycle through the eons. Hence Brahman here is not a being, it is the ground of all that exists, and this universe passes through cycles of creation and dissolution because of its own nature. It neither wills it itself, nor is there anything else outside of it to make it go through the cycles.

One such cycle of evolution is called a day of Brahman. Such a day is said to equal 4,320 million years, or four billion human years. This estimate is the same as the estimated age of the universe up to ten years ago, although at present the universe is said to be about ten to twelve billion years old. This is followed by the "night" of Brahman, or *pralay*, of an equal length, when the Brahman remains in an un-manifested form. Then another day of evolution begins.

The Buddhist view of the origin of the universe is different. For them, the universe has always existed in this state of "dependent arising" (*pratitya samutpada*). This position is the same as the "steady state" theory of the universe.

The essential difference between the Buddhist and the Advaitic views can be seen as the difference between a digital and an analog world. "Digital" is, for example, the flow of time in a digital watch, with the time in figures, where changes in time occur in jumps or multiples. "Analog" is the flow in a watch with hands, where there is continuous steady flow.

In Buddhism, everything is seen to be composed of discontinuous, discrete particles. Even the flow of time is seen as merely a stream of discontinuous moments, which add together. Consciousness also is a stream of individual flashes of thoughts and sensations. In Advaitism, on the other hand, there is a steady flow of time and space; the universe is a seamless whole and is connected in entirety, not in itself but because of the presence of an absolute behind it.

Science appears in some ways to indicate the answer in favor of "analog" existence. Facts like the interchangeability of matter and energy and "no empty space" would all logically indicate a seamless stream of existence. On the other hand, there is as yet no theory for any "absolute" behind it all. Hence this question remains to be answered.

The one aspect of our existence that has generated the greatest amount of debate, whether among religions, in philosophy, or in science is consciousness. Consciousness explains who we are; it specifies us not only as an order of existence, as living objects, but it also marks us out on the individual level. The "I" of each of us is this consciousness.

It is difficult to define consciousness. But on a simple basis, it can be considered as awareness, awareness of both the self and that outside the self—the non-self, as it were. As a result of this awareness, living objects can utilize the environment for their survival. Consciousness is also characterized by learning behavior, and higher levels of consciousness are determined by corresponding higher capacities to learn.

Explaining consciousness has been one of the main considerations of religious theories. Most religions offer the explanation that consciousness is a god-given gift and is the property of an independent entity in itself, the soul. The soul is a higher entity and merely inhabits the body and runs it, and consciousness has no connection to the body or the universe as such.

On the other hand, modern science is firmly of the opinion that consciousness does not demand such an extra-natural explanation and is directly related to the functioning of the brain, although how exactly is something that we are yet to discover. There seems to be no reason to assume, at least until now, that there is any luminous object like the soul that makes humans conscious. Much of the brain is known, and we are even beginning to find out not just the centers for the senses, but even the centers for different forms of emotions, analysis, and so on. The brain, as is easily seen, is affected by chemicals like alcohol and drugs, and these can change aspects of our consciousness, like moods. All these show that consciousness is directly related to the human brain, and there is no supernatural entity that is the basis of consciousness.

On a strictly neurological interpretation, the brain is composed of billions of brain cells, which are intricately interconnected by nerves. The neurons are constantly sending electrical signals to each other, and these signals carry *information* from one neuron to the others. Each neuron is in turn receiving signals from many other neurons, and depending on the signals it is receiving, it sends out its own signals. Thus there is a continuous exchange of information within the brain, a constant "*pool* of information."

On the basis of our present knowledge of the world, it seems reasonably safe to assume that the activity of the brain, which generates individual consciousness, is this continuous exchange of information within itself, the "information *pool*." Information about the outside world is generated through the sensory organs. The sensory organs convert the world outside into streams of signals, which carry information to the brain. When we "see" something, for example, the eye does not send the picture itself to the brain. The signals from the eye are converted into information that is coded into electrical signals; this information is then fed into the "pool of information," and this eventually is interpreted in the pool as the picture.

What is most puzzling about this is that there is nothing here that is "intelligent," that does any "conscious" function. The individual neurons cannot be said to do any "intelligent" processing or analysis, they cannot be said to have understood anything of the signals they receive. They are merely mechanical transmitters, which on receiving certain signals mechanically transmit out other signals in their turn.

Somehow, during this intense flux of information, in ways that are still very far from being understood, our individual consciousness is manifested. Our consciousness is not in the brain cells, the nerves, or the electrical signals being transmitted in the nerves, it is in the pool of "information flux" that is being generated in it. Rather, we might say, our consciousness *is* this "information flux." Hence it is not the matter or the electric charge of the brain that is important, it is this "information flux" or "information pool" that determines who we are.

Defining individual consciousness as an "information flux" does not go against the Advaitic understanding of consciousness; rather it complements Advaitic metaphysics. Advaita also interprets individual consciousness as a part of relative existence only, and hence as part of the world. Advaita recognizes two forms of consciousness, the absolute consciousness and the individual consciousness. Advaita recognizes our individual consciousness as being very much on the plane of this world.

All individual consciousness is limited, transitory, and ill-defined, just as all material existence in the world. All consciousness in the world is a particularized, limited part of the absolute. It is analogous to the way the existence of matter is explained as being on two planes, the absolute existence of Brahman and the particularized existence of the material world. Here too there is the absolute consciousness of Brahman and the individualized consciousness on the plane of the world.

Hence Advaita would have no difficulty in accepting that the individual consciousness is a part of worldly existence of matter and energy, and is on the same level with it. Hence Advaita would accept easily that individual consciousness is generated in the brain.

Only it would say that the individual consciousness is only a limited part of the absolute consciousness of Brahman. Absolute consciousness is eternal, indivisible, unchanging, and unknowable. Individual consciousness is particularized consciousness, a manifested form of consciousness, changing, individualized, and transitory.

Our consciousness is a part of the phenomena of the universe, no matter how we define it. It is certainly not something that is separate from the rest of the universe. The Brahman lies as the basis of everything in the universe. It cannot be that one dimension of existence, the material aspect, exists because of Brahman, while the other dimension, consciousness, exists by itself. Both are part of the same universe. Hence, necessarily, the Brahman must lie as the basis of consciousness also.

In Advaita, there are two planes or levels of existence: the absolute plane of Brahman and the relative plane of this universe. Again, on the relative plane, the universe is considered to have three dimensions or domains of existence: *sat*, *chit*, and *ananda*, or existence, consciousness, and bliss. These are the three dimensions or domains in which Brahman is manifested in the universe.

The universe exists in these three dimensions. These three dimensions, intertwined like the strands in a rope or cloth, form the universe. The material dimension is the dimension that we see around us, the matter-energy of the universe. The consciousness dimension is what we experience as our own individual consciousness, and also see in others. Bliss is the third dimension, which is experienced in Yoga and mystical experiences. So the universe has this threefold existence, and all three dimensions exist simultaneously as potential at all points of the universe, although they may not be manifested. These three domains are the three modes in which the Brahman is expressed in the universe.

An analogy, although imperfect, would be the white light composed of red, green, and blue beams. All three colors exist intermingled and simultaneously in the same space and time, but they all exist in their own dimensions or domains, in this case in different domains of wavelengths. Ultimately they can be traced back to the common origin of the source of light. So also matter and consciousness exist in the universe in their own dimensions, or "wavelengths," of manifestation.

> *Let thy mind with the mind, let thy breath with the breath*
> *(of the Gods be united).*
> *Be this offering rich in ghee pleasing to the gods; hail!*
> *May Indra's expiration be set in every limb;*
> *May Indra's inspiration be in every limb.*

O god Tvastr, let mind be united for thee,
When ye that are various become of one form!

—Sama Veda, 1.3.10

When we define consciousness in modern terms to be an "information flux," then also we see that this information flux has a different dimension or sphere of existence from matter. This information flux is supported by matter, but it is not dependent on a particular piece of matter, as it could be supported or generated by many different types of matter. It could be supported by silicon chips, by mechanical machines, or by biological forms like the brain. The information flux in the brain, for example, would have worked just as well if the signals carrying the information were pulses of light instead of electrical potentials in nerves.

It is logical to suppose that if we could "read" all the information being generated and passed on between the neurons in our brain, and then create an artificial circuit using silicon or some such device that is exactly the same as the brain circuit, and then fed this entire information to it and activated it, we would have a duplicate human consciousness. The electrical potentials by themselves are not important in the flux; it is the *information*, which is carried in the sequence of their transmission, which is vital. The information exists, as it were, as an independent entity and is only carried by the electrical signals.

"Information" can be said to exist both dependently and independently of matter-energy. It is dependent because it depends on existence itself; it would not exist if there was no other existence in the universe. On the other hand, it can exist potentially with any form of existence that is manifested from the absolute. At the same time, whenever there is existence of matter, it means that, simultaneously, there is existence of information about that matter. For example, if a rock exists, there exists information about it, such as its mass, velocity, shape, number, and so forth. This information is defined in relation to other information systems, just as the physical properties of the rock are defined against other physical particles. Thus consciousness, or information flux, may be said to be potentially able to be manifest whenever there is any manifestation of existence in the universe.

Hence it is dependent not on any individual manifestation of matter but on manifestation itself, and both matter-energy and information are, because of their very nature, always manifested simultaneously. Of course, although all matter has information tagged along with it, it is only when the matter is organized in a way that information also becomes organized that we have consciousness, as in the nerve matter of life.

Hence although it coexists with matter and energy, it is a separate aspect, a separate domain of existence, apart from the material aspect of the existence of the signals. Thus consciousness (the information flux) coexists with the brain but has a different dimension of existence than the *matter* of the brain. This is the same as the Advaitic concept where consciousness, or chit, is a different dimension of manifestation that coexists with sat, or material existence. In this way, the modern concept of consciousness agrees well with the Advaitic concepts.

If we call the individual consciousness an information flux, then we may call the absolute consciousness of Brahman the "universal information field," containing information (i.e., awareness of everything), and of which this individual awareness is but a small, dynamic, ill-defined part. Brahman has in it not only the potential for all of material existence, but also the potential for all of the information about this existence. Individual information flux can exist as an entity only because this universal field of information, or Brahman, underlies everything in the universe. This universal information lies at the root, as the basis of all individualized flux

On one side, we may say, the generalized "existence" of Brahman is particularized to the individual material "existence" of objects like the matter-energy of the brain. On the other side, we may say that the generalized "universal information" or "absolute consciousness" of Brahman is particularized to the individual "information flux" or "individual consciousness" of living beings. Each individual information flux or each individual consciousness is like a wave on the ocean of the "consciousness dimension" of Brahman, just as matter is like a wave on the "material dimension."

Here it must be emphasized that we ascribe terms like absolute existence and absolute consciousness to Brahman only to define individual existence and consciousness. Brahman, however, does not have these different aspects such as absolute consciousness and absolute existence; it is the same indivisible Brahman that qualified in one way gives rise to material existence and qualified in another way gives rise to individual consciousness.

Brahman is the universal field out of which are generated individual matter, consciousness, and bliss. When we are talking of matter being generated from this universal field, we call it absolute matter; when we are talking of consciousness being generated, we call it absolute consciousness, and so on.

The claim of Yoga is simply that in samadhi, we become capable of accessing this universal information. Normally we identify ourselves with the material dimension, our bodies. On further contemplation, we identify with our thoughts and feelings, the consciousness dimension. Through the practice of Yoga, we can learn to identify with the bliss dimension. But it is only through samadhi, the final mystical experience, that we learn to identify with the base of everything, Brahman itself.

Death means merely that the information being realized in our brains ceases to be played on, but this individualized information was but a small, limited part of the infinite information, in which the information continues to exist. Hence this information does not die out or cease to exist. It continues not as an individual anymore, but as part of the infinite, dissolved in the infinite of Brahman, as it were.

The story is told of a salt doll that wanted to measure the depth of the sea. But as she went into it, she herself dissolved and became a part of the sea. In the same way, during the mystical experience or in death our "individual consciousness" dissolves or expands into the infinite field of Brahman.

A confounding factor in our understanding of consciousness has been the development of computers. From the way computers react to us with their audiovisual and analytical abilities, we seem to feel it is an almost human media interacting with us. But seeing consciousness in today's computers will be like the child believing that there are humans inside radios who make the sounds. They are still only reflections of the human consciousness. But as time progresses, computers may evolve to become more and more similar to humans, and finally acquire learning capacity. It seems certain that, with further progress in the science, eventually a working form of something that we can call consciousness will be generated.

Even considering that there could be the presence of an artificial consciousness is often disturbing, because consciousness seems to be such a unique thing to us. For traditional religions, it would be a shattering development, as it would mean the final nail in the coffin to all their concepts of souls and god. But of course, consciousness has never been a sole human reserve. It has always existed outside the human brain, in animals, birds, and more.

In Advaita, generation of an artificial consciousness would not contradict any of its philosophy regarding the universe. Consciousness in Advaita is inherent in the universe, a dimension of existence of the universe, and hence it only needs the proper conditions for its manifestation. If consciousness is indeed a part of the natural and known universe, then there is no logical bar to our creating consciousness. This has already happened accidentally once during evolution. Presence of a "conscious" computer would only mean that humans have learnt to exploit this natural capacity of the universe, to make manifest what was always potential in it.

If we call consciousness an information flux, then we could say that in computers, man has only learnt to access the dimension of information that is inherent everywhere in the universe. In a computer we have learnt to arrange matter-energy in such a way that the information dimension is also manifested in that aspect. Moreover, this information dimension or consciousness dimension can be manifested not just in one way, but in various ways utilizing matter-energy in many different ways, as in the early mechanical computers, the present silicon computers, and DNA computers of the future. We have only learnt now to make manifest what had already been done earlier during evolution.

Of course, in our present computers, the information that is generated and fed is relevant only to us; it is not self-relevant— that is, it is not relevant to the computer itself. Hence the present day computers cannot be called conscious in that sense. But once a computer acquires learning capacity, the information will become relevant to it, and it will be able to utilize information to change its responses. At this point, computers could be considered "conscious" in the way that we understand consciousness.

In fact, the generation of consciousness in ways other than the biological, as in computers, will indicate the truth of the Advaitic view that the universe exists everywhere in these three dimensions of materiality, consciousness, and bliss. That consciousness can be manifested in so many ways and in so many different conditions of matter and energy shows that consciousness is a basic property of all existence. That there can be so many different types of consciousness shows that there must be a common "ground" of consciousness.

Discovery of life on other planets and alien consciousness will only show up this universal character of consciousness, and will lend further support to the Advaitic view. All these different forms of consciousness—human consciousness, lion consciousness, virus consciousness, computer consciousness, and even space-alien consciousness—can then be seen as but different limitations of the same absolute field of Brahman.

All these theories are only logical arguments at present, and we may wonder if we will ever know the truth behind consciousness. Our knowledge of consciousness today is very limited, and our means of exploring it even more so. But science, as it has changed everything else, is likely to change this aspect too. We are likely to know more and more by advancement in two main fields: medical science and computers. Many things that once seemed mysterious and beyond human understanding are now considered quite simple. Similarly, we will perhaps soon one day understand what exactly consciousness is about and how it works. Then perhaps we will be able to solve the final question of Advaita—whether there lies an absolute consciousness beyond this or not. Hence it is likely that the Advaita position on consciousness too will be settled on way or the other soon.

Arise, awake, and learn by approaching the excellent ones.
The wise ones describe that path to be as impassable as a
razor's edge, which, when sharpened, is difficult to tread on.

—Katha Upanishad I.iii.14

In many other ways we can see some of the concepts of the Upanishads to be remarkably similar to modern science. The theory of evolution is one such argument, which shook up virtually the entire world of religion and destroyed much of it. But even as other religions were struggling to try to make some sense of it, we find Swami Vivekananda in the eighteenth century welcoming it and using it in his speeches to vindicate Advaitism.

The methods used by the sages of the Upanishads were not scientific, in the modern sense of the term. The sages studied the inner phenomenon using our self-awareness to arrive at conclusions regarding the world as a whole. This was the method of study used everywhere prior to the sixteenth century, with some rare exceptions. Such methods invariably led to wide differences due to subjectivity, and the conclusions are not subject to being contradicted or repeated. Hence there were usually many defects in the details.

But modern science uses our external awareness—the study of external objects—to arrive at the knowledge of the world. This study allows for objectiveness and experimentation, which fulfill our rational impulses. But the main theories in the Upanishads regarding the world were quite remarkably the same as that of modern physics. In fact, Advaitism may be said to have preceded present scientific knowledge in some spheres by several thousand years.

Advaitism provides a firm philosophical support for scientific study. In Advaitism, beyond this world lies the absolute, and further and greater knowledge of the world will lead us to the absolute. Hence there is a goal for all knowledge, all science and arts and every human endeavor in Advaitism, and this is to bring us nearer and nearer to the true knowledge. In Advaitism, it is said, the more our true knowledge, the closer we will be led to the absolute. This in the Upanishads is the concept of *vidya* and *avidya*.

Vidya is the intellectual conception of the truth. *Vidya*, in Advaitic terms, is the conception of the absolute Brahman, and all other conceptions of the truth are false, or avidya. Science, along with logic, aesthetics, and so forth, has this important role in that it brings us to this intellectual conception of the truth. Advaita does not accept that the truth is beyond intellectual conception, only that it is indescribable in terms of our human experience. But Advaita says that merely having this intellectual conception is not enough. It is only the first step, and for the spiritual goal we have to proceed beyond this for the mystical experience, an intense and total awareness of the absolute, which is far beyond a bare intellectual conception. Hence vidya or an intellectual conception of the truth alone is not the goal of spirituality, and this is what makes Advaita a religion and not just philosophical speculation.

The importance of Advaitism lies in its suitability for our modern ethos. At the present age, people in general are not willing to accept a religion that contradicts our reason or scientific knowledge. Religions based entirely on dogmas do not find ready acceptance. The increasing refinement and awareness of human society has also made us more aware of other peoples and the need to respect and follow other religions. We find it difficult to accept religious dogmas that demean other gods and call our own god the highest. The modern person is increasingly taking to religious forms that absorb the best ideals from all religions, and there is greater respect and awareness of other religions than ever before.

Advaitism is important in this context because of its scientific basis. There is no call to obey dogmas, rather aspirants are advised to think after hearing, to confirm and argue within themselves until they are satisfied with what they have heard. Only then are we to follow the teachings. First hear, then think, then act—this is the great method of religion in the Upanishads. This is something that no other religion has dared to advise its followers. Again, among all religions, Hinduism has always been at the forefront of religious tolerance. "The truth is one, the wise call it by many names."

It is a settled truism in Hinduism since ancient times that all gods are but different names of the same truth. Hinduism has also long been amenable to a "mix-and-match" form of religious observance. In the Yoga sutras of Patanjali, the form on which the aspirant is to meditate is not fixed; a large number of forms is given, and the aspirant is advised to pick any form "which arouses respect." Hence other religious paths can easily access the strength of Yoga. This essential modern spirit of the Upanishads is the force behind the continuing strength of Advaita to the present day.

Part Two

Karmakanda: Actions

9

Mysticism
and the Four Yogas

This plaint of the flute is fire, not mere air.
Let him who lacks this fire be accounted dead!
'Tis the fire of love that inspires the flute,
'Tis the ferment of love that possesses the wine.
The flute is the confidant of all unhappy lovers;
Yea, its strains lay bare my inmost secrets.
Who hath seen a poison and an antidote like the flute?

—Muhammad Rumi, Book 1

All aspects of Hinduism ultimately boil down to mysticism, which is the goal of the religion. Mysticism means contact with the absolute within the living body (although the word is frequently used as a kind of synonym for any mystery connected with spiritual matters). This absolute may be understood in any form, from the personal god of dualism to the absolute Brahman of Advaita, but the defining moment is a contact with this higher truth.

Of course, mysticism is sought not just in Hinduism, but also in practically all religions, including Christianity and Islam. In other religions, though, the mystical experience is not the goal of the orthodox doctrines, and mystics are often considered rebels—that is, when they are not persecuted outright. The goal in such primarily dualistic religions is to live according to the book so as to ensure reaching heaven in the hereafter; true religion lies in living a good life as defined in the doctrines.

But in Hinduism, the goal of religion is *solely* this contact with the truth, and until this is achieved, the spiritual quest is considered incomplete. All other things are considered secondary to this supreme end, and no performance of religious duties can be a substitute. Hence the Upanishads declare, alone among all religious texts, that they are not the end of religion, and the truly religious must go beyond them in their spiritual quest. These strikingly daring words—where the religious texts themselves declare that true religion lies beyond them, and that they are only a pointer—have come to define the Hindu spiritual life, with its tolerance and broadmindedness.

The understanding of mystical experience flows logically from the Advaitic understanding of the nature of the world and Brahman. In Advaitic metaphysics, there are two planes of existence: the absolute plane of Brahman and the relative plane of our world. At the base of relative existence is the absolute Brahman. But this relative world is an undefined state, and it exists only because it has Brahman at the base. All existence ultimately flows from Brahman, and that which we see as discrete existence is shadowy and unformed. Hence the true essence of everything is Brahman, and if we shift away that which is untrue, we will come to Brahman. Ramakrishna described this as removing the green mossy layer of a pond to reveal the clear water beneath it.

The relative existence, the universe of our everyday experience, exists in three dimensions: the material dimension, consciousness dimension, and bliss dimension. Our personal existence in the relative world is also in these three dimensions. When we consider what we mean by "I," at first thought we may say, "our bodies." This is the material dimension of our "I." But on deeper reflection, we would say "our individual consciousness." On further meditation, we can exist in the bliss dimension, when we will not know any individual consciousness but exist only in and as bliss.

The Upanishads define bliss to be our true identity. Bliss is the purest and most natural state of our existence. It is when our consciousness is drawn outward that we are diverted from this bliss. This definition of our true identity is the lynchpin of all Upanishadic mysticism, and the goal of Yoga is to stop the outward diversion and regain this natural state of supreme happiness. But even beyond this is the final experience of mysticism, when we will exist only as the absolute Brahman.

The individual consciousness in the Upanishads is considered to be a complex of "I"-thoughts and sensations. The organ of mind is called the *Antahkarna*, and it is said to have three modes: the ego, or "I-ness"; the *Buddhi*, or the deciding part; and the *Manas*, or the mind, or the part that sends its sensations on to the Buddhi. *Citta*, the mind-stuff, constitutes all these three just as atoms constitute the material world. This is the psychological interpretation of individual consciousness in Hinduism, and it is accepted by all streams of thought. It is important to note here that the ego, or "I-ness," is considered to be a part of the complex and there is no independent or separate "I"; the entire complex of "I"-ness-thoughts-sensations stands together and constitutes the individual consciousness.

Again, this individual consciousness is considered to have only a shadowy, ill-defined existence, and it can exist only because there is the Brahman at the base. In Advaitism, we are not the "I" thoughts and sensations; we are actually the unlimited Brahman, and it is only because of our delusion that the "I" thoughts and sensations appear to us to be our identity. Hence if we "clear" away this individual consciousness, there will exist only the Brahman. This is the explanation of the mystical experience in Advaita. All mystical efforts are only an attempt to control and "clear" away the individual consciousness; this will expose what lies at the root, the absolute Brahman.

Since individual consciousness consists of the complex of "I"-ness, thoughts, and sensations, what is needed is to control any or all of these factors and the whole complex will fall away by itself. This is how Advaita explains why there are so many different ways of attaining mystical experiences. They all ultimately lead to dissolution of the individual consciousness, and this exposes the absolute behind it. The same process at the heart of all mysticism explains the similarity of such experiences everywhere, while differences in the levels of achieving this dissolution explain the disparities.

Thus, in Raja Yoga the suppression is attained by psychological methods alone, through intense concentration and conscious attempts at suppressing thoughts. In Jnana Yoga it is attained by meditation, in Karma Yoga by achieving a state of indifference, and in Bhakti Yoga by intense absorption in the beloved.

In modern knowledge, consciousness has often been understood as an information flux, an intense whirlpool of information being circulated in the brain, resulting in consciousness. This explanation fits in very well with the metaphysical and psychological theories of Advaita. In the modern explanation, the "information flux" is not a part of the material world, although it is supported by it. It cannot be called simply a product of the physical structure that supports it, because the same information can be transmitted in other ways with the same effect. Hence we may well say that the "information flux" exists in a different dimension to the material world.

This is the same as the Advaitic view of the different dimensions of existence of consciousness and the material world. But in Advaitic terms, nothing in this world can exist in itself; it exists only because there is an absolute at the base. It cannot be that one dimension of existence, the material aspect, exists because of Brahman while the other dimension, consciousness, exists by itself. Both are part of the same universe. Hence if the "information flux" exists, there must be an "absolute information field" to support it. In that case, we can understand mysticism as nothing more than the merger of the individual "information flux" in this "absolute information field," or Brahman.

Advaita recognizes three states of our individual consciousness: the waking, dream, and dreamless sleep. Beyond this is the fourth stage, the stage of super-consciousness, also called *Turiya*. It is when the mind is in this state that it attains the bliss of samadhi.

Normally our minds are constantly moving outwards—that is, toward the objects of our thoughts and sensations, the world. This is called *pravritti*, like an enlarging circle of ripples in a pond. But when we can make the mind move in an inward movement, or *nivritti*, the mind becomes gradually stilled; ultimately, when it reaches a single point (that is, our individuality becomes suppressed to only a point of existence), it achieves the state of bliss. Bliss is not considered simply a part of individual consciousness but a different dimension of existence altogether. This is because what we understand by consciousness is the complex of "I-ness," our thoughts and sensations, and because the state of bliss exists only when this complex becomes infinitely small, it is not considered just another state of consciousness.

But even a higher state than this exists, the state of complete extermination of all individuality. This is the state of final samadhi, Nirvikalpa Samadhi. This is beyond even bliss, and what is experienced in this state cannot be described. This is the goal of all Advaitism.

The state of samadhi, or mystical union, is not a single state in Advaita but has several stages. Different stages give rise to varied experiences, as a result of which we have diverse views of the nature of the absolute and the world. Advaita says there are three stages of mystical experience: dualistic, qualified monistic, and monistic.

In the dualistic form of mysticism, there is no loss or diminution of the individual personality in mystical experience. The individual consciousness itself comes into contact with the divine. This is seen when God and humans are considered to be two separate existences. God created humans, and so there can be no equivalence between the two. Both retain their identity, but the person comes face-to-face with, is in direct contact with, and is able to "see" the infinite truth. Of this quality are the descriptions of "visions" of angels or even God given by saints of dualistic religions.

Next comes the qualified monistic form of mysticism, in which humans have a relationship to God wherein they are the part and God is the whole. Here the individual consciousnesses of the persons who undergo the mystical experience realize the great truth and lose the differentiation that kept them from realizing that they were part of the truth. They come into contact with the divine and feel themselves a part of it. But the individual expression is not lost completely.

Last is the Advaitic expression, in which all individual expression is lost and the individual personality dies out, and only the absolute Brahman is experienced. Advaita explains the differences in these different perceptions of mysticism as the differences to which the individual personality is obliterated. In dualism, when the individual personality is not wiped out but only becomes very fine, as it were, then we see the glimmering of the absolute through the transparent vestige of our personality, and see it as the divine in accordance with the view retained by this last stage of our thoughts. In qualified monism, there is further loss of our personality; we feel at one with the absolute, but still retain the faintest traces of our personality and hence feel the relation of part and whole. But in the Advaitic experience there is no personality left at all, and there is only the pure Brahman shining through.

The analogy given for the mystical experience in Hinduism is the lakebed seen through the ripples. Here the lakebed is the presence of Brahman, which lies at the root of our consciousness. The ripples in the lake waters are our thoughts and emotions, which cloud up the waters so that the pure Brahman is not manifested. Another analogy is the dirty mirror that does not reflect the sun until we clear up the dirt of our thoughts, and the sun then becomes manifest. Again, it is also described as seeing the sun through a hole in a piece of cloth, which becomes clearer and clearer the more we enlarge the hole. The basic point is the same, that the more we control our thoughts, the clearer the Brahman is manifested.

> *O my heart! The Supreme Spirit, the great Master, is near you, wake, oh wake!*
> *Run to the feet of your Beloved, for the Lord stands near your head.*
> *You have slept for unnumbered ages; this morning will you not wake?*
>
> —Kabir, 3.20

The accounts of mystics often vary widely; for example, Christian saints would describe a vision of God or an angel differently than Islamic saints. In Advaita, these different experiences are explained to be due to the differences in the paths followed that lead toward the same absolute. The different mystical paths may be seen as spokes of a wheel going toward the same center. The further away we are from the center, the greater the "personality content" of the mystical experience, and the more the difference in the accounts. As we approach nearer to the absolute, the accounts of mystics become more and more similar, and they finally merge when the pure absolute is obtained.

The dualistic experience is considered to be further away, and the dualistic mystics see the absolute in terms of the god that they define in their religion. The next stage is that of the qualified monist, and depending on the nearness to the center, the accounts become more and more similar. As in their metaphysical theories, so also in their mystical experiences; qualified monists describe a wide range of experiences, from the purely dualistic to an almost Advaitic one among the more monistic teachers.

The final stage of all mystical experience in Hinduism is Nirvikalpa Samadhi. In this stage, there is not the slightest vestige of personality, and the mystic experiences the absolute, unqualified reality. Even existence, consciousness, and bliss are still qualities and hence only reflections of our consciousness. But Brahman in its absolute stage cannot have any qualities at all, and in Nirvikalpa Samadhi, Brahman is experienced as being beyond even these qualities. The absolute here is seen as something that lies beyond all relativistic conceptions, and there is no sufficient description to meet it. The monistic mystics of *all* religions—Christianity, Islam, Zen Buddhism, and Advaitism—describe this stage, although in the other religions their accounts have been sidelined from the mainstream religion.

These three types of mystical experiences can be found not just in Hinduism but also in other religions like Christianity and Islam. In Christianity, the mystics are not considered to be part of the orthodox religion. The main doctrines of Christianity do not support the mystical experience, and it is mainly a practical religion with the goal of leading a good life so as to finally reach heaven in the hereafter. But despite this, mystics have been an important source of inspiration to Christians everywhere.

Among Christian mystics also, we find these three types of mystical experiences. The dualistic is the most common form of the Christian mystical writings and is the most widely accepted by the official church. Dualistic interpretations range from visions of Jesus to contact with the divine being, which in Christian terms is defined as the Holy Ghost, the intermediary between God and humans and the aspect of God that is accessible to us.

But there are many other mystics who showed a clear qualified monistic interpretation, and described contact with the divine, which was of the same nature as the self, and merger of the self with this truth. Again there were mystics, mainly the later ones, whose writings showed a clear monistic truth, and who spoke of a complete merger in which there was no differentiation or self.

Similarly, this threefold expression of mysticism is seen in Islam as well. Islamic mystics are called Sufis, and the position of the Muslim orthodoxy toward all mystics was more or less the same as in Christianity. But here, too, Sufis, with their message of universal harmony, had the same strong influence as in Christianity. The earliest Sufis described a dualistic position with relation to Allah, and spoke of visions or a feeling of nearness toward Allah.

But we also find descriptions of a more intimate relation to him as in qualified monism among later Sufis. Finally, we also find a monistic expression of mysticism among some schools of Sufis, mainly in India.

Thus the mystical experience is a universal one and is held on broadly similar terms by all religions and cultures. Advaita is able to harmonize all mystical experiences and show the universal truth, which lies beyond them. Hence the Upanishads declare "God is one, the wise call it by various names." This is the highest expression of religious harmony to be found anywhere. In Hinduism, there is no claim to an exclusive god; rather, it recognizes that there is one ultimate truth, and it is only we who call it different names. All religions and all mystical experiences lead to this same truth. This realization is the basis for the spiritual tolerance of Hinduism.

The truth of the unqualified absolute, the end stage of all mystical experience, is not particular to Advaitists; mystics from all religions have arrived at the same experience. Dualistic and qualified monistic experiences are more common. But in every religion, there have always been mystics who have crossed these stages and arrived at the final stage, in which there is complete loss of personality and the person realizes the truth of monism, that there is only one absolute truth. This has been realized by monistic mystics of Christianity and Islam. Zen and Yogachara mysticism also aim for the same monistic end, the realization of a single truth. However, the question might arise that, if the same monistic absolute is encountered by all, then why are there different paths leading to monism and different metaphysical conceptions of the absolute?

The answer, according to Advaitism, is that these conceptions are formed only when the absolute is sought to be described in terms of our world, in terms of our everyday experiences. The essence of the absolute is that it is without qualities. It is qualities like hardness, redness, shape, and so on that bind us and give rise to our discrete existence. We can only comprehend something that is bound and differentiated by such qualities.

The arguments between, say, Advaitists and Zen Buddhists relate only to the intellectual conception of this absolute. Zen mystics also try to achieve the state of "suchness" of the mind, in which the mind becomes free of its personality content and remains in its essential nature. Thus Yogachara and Zen use the same Yogic formulae to approach the mystical experience as in Advaitism. The same unqualified absolute is experienced by Advaitists, Zen Buddhists. and non-dualistic mystics from all religions and cultures. But in trying to describe something that is by nature indescribable, they have to see it through the prism of their philosophy, and hence in the elaborations of the goal, we find differences in their positions. The Madhyamikas also experience the same absolute, but because of their philosophy of absolute nihilism, they describe the essential "indescribability" of the absolute in negative terms and take it as *shunya*.

Such arguments are important only in the course of forming our intellectual *concepts*; they do not make any difference in the ultimate *experience* of religion. The descriptions of the experiences in mysticism are remarkably similar among both Zen Buddhists and Advaitists, as well as monistic mystics of other religions. The initial stages of all mystical experience are different because they approach through different paths. But they ultimately converge on the same absolute. So as the mystical experience becomes deeper, experience also becomes similar. Because of this, the descriptions also converge.

Once we accept the non-dualistic absolute as our spiritual goal, the question of which path to follow is only a question of philosophy; it does not make any difference to our practical experience of religion. We must accept the path that most appeals to us and satisfies our needs. What we choose will depend on our personal predilections, but in general, the path that appears the most harmonious and logical to us will have the strongest appeal.

The dualistic precepts of religions like Christianity and Islam are not fully amenable to monistic thought. Non-dualistic mystics in these religions could not be said to be true to their essential doctrines. The Zen and Yogachara philosophies also, with their precept of extreme solipsism in which it says the world is only a dream of the mind, proffer a strange metaphysics. Besides, these forms of Buddhism, with their essentially pessimistic view of negating life, which are also opposed to science, logic, the arts, and social feelings, cannot give coherence to life. It is in this context that the philosophy of Advaitism, which harmonizes the absolute and the world, and at the same time is extremely logical and rational, has its importance for all spiritual seekers.

The mysticism of Theravada Buddhism is of a different order. In this there is no experience of a higher state, because there *is* no higher state. Instead the mystical experience in Theravada comprises a complete identification with the *knowledge* preached by the Buddha, where the world is known in all its aspects and is seen as a relative reality only without any absolute as its basis. Thus in Theravada, there is no higher *state* to experience, but only a higher *knowledge* to acquire. Shunya cannot be experienced because it is not there. Theravada Buddhists emphatically reject any claims of knowing Shunya or experiencing Shunya, because by definition it cannot be known or experienced. Shunya is thus a doctrinal definition only, and one believes in it only on the basis of the teachings of the Buddha or the logical arguments given for it by his followers.

Advaita cannot be reconciled with Theravada mysticism, just as it finds the experiences of dualism and qualified monism unsatisfactory. The knowledge of Advaitism and Theravada Buddhism are of two diametrically opposite realities. In the Advaitic view, Theravada Buddhism is a doctrinal teaching only. There is no true mystical experience in Theravada Buddhism, only a complete identification of the aspirant with its teachings.

The Buddha emphatically rejected all mystical experiences as unnecessary and considered the process of trying to acquire them as dangerous. His path was aimed at removing the sorrows of humankind, and for this it was not necessary to search for something beyond the world. All that was necessary was to have an incontrovertible belief in what he taught, and once the aspirant acquired this belief, he would acquire the tranquility of Buddhahood. This is not the mystical experience of Advaitism or Zen, and the great defect is that the teachings themselves are not put to the test; the aspirant only acquires them. Theravada Buddhism would therefore be considered in Advaitism only as a set of beliefs, which depends on the faith of the aspirants, and not a true religion in that it does not give the aspirant any direct experience of the truth.

> *How strict and detached were the lives the holy hermits led in the desert! What long and grave temptations they suffered! How often were they beset by the enemy! What frequent and ardent prayers they offered to God! What rigorous fasts they observed! How great their zeal and their love for spiritual perfection! How brave their fight!*
>
> —Thomas à Kempis, *The Imitation of Christ*

Though there are often intellectual differences in categorizing their experiences, we can undeniably feel the throb of a universal truth in the writings of mystics throughout the world. The descriptions of what they experience in that state is uniform, even when what they theorize from it differs. Through studies of writings of various mystics around the world, some common points relating to mystical experiences may be identified.

The noetic quality: Persons undergoing the mystical experience have the conviction that they have acquired a true knowledge, that they have realized the fundamental truth of the world and have gained an insight into the reality behind all phenomena.

Feeling of bliss: This is also one of the universal mystical expressions. The mystics feel a total sense of bliss, of happiness and joy, and this is of an overwhelming intensity.

Sense of sacredness: The mystics feel a deep sense of awe in front of the absolute reality that they face directly and feel an intense sense of spiritual fulfillment.

Transcendence of time and space: The mystics feel liberated from time and space, and they always describe the absolute as being beyond the boundaries of both time and space.

Union of opposites: Mystics also describe the absolute as being beyond the opposites—for example, beyond being conscious and unconscious, infinitely large and infinitely small, and so on. No such logical parameters of our everyday life apply to the absolute.

Indescribability: The absolute is always said to be indescribable. This follows from the fact that the absolute is beyond the parameters of our everyday world, and therefore our language is inadequate to describe it. But descriptions are still made with metaphors and analogies, and also by expanding our use of language.

Transiency: The person does not remain in the mystical state for long and soon comes back into the temporal world, where the sense of non-duality is lost.

Positive changes: After the experience, the person exhibits feelings of love and oneness with all and also attains deep wisdom.

The defining description of the mystical experience is that it is a state of bliss. This is perhaps the most universal point made by mystics throughout all ages and cultures, including the Upanishads. The most pure state of our consciousness, the undifferentiated state, is described as a blissful state. Normally our consciousness is in a restless state of a thousand different emotions and feelings. But all emotions and feelings in the Advaitic view proceed from the state of bliss. Because the mind is restless, this state of bliss is distorted, and we experience our different emotions. But in the mystical state, the mind is said to be in utter peace and unmoving. In this state, the pure state of consciousness is experienced, and it is then in a state of bliss.

It is important to understand that "bliss" here is not just used in the abstract sense to convey a state of tranquility. It is an actual emotion and is the same as the happiness and pleasure that we feel in our daily lives, only it is many times more intense. It would perhaps be more appropriate to call it "ecstasy," much like the ecstasy we feel at particular moments in our lives, as when we achieve success in love, in our career, or even during sex.

In the Upanishads, this bliss is directly compared to the happiness of social life. The Upanishads first take the image of a person, a king, who is all-powerful, has no worries, and has practically all his wishes granted. The Upanishads then raise the picture of the happiness of such a person, then go on to say how many thousands and thousands of times more intense than this is the happiness of the state of samadhi. The intention here is to show that the bliss, or ecstasy, of samadhi is not different from the happiness we experience in our daily lives, but is a million times more intense and pure than this. In this way, the Upanishads show us that the ecstasy of samadhi is not something alien to us, but that in the happiest moments of our lives, we get just the faintest whiff of this richness.

But the final stage of Yoga, the Nirvikalpa Samadhi, is beyond even this bliss. The individual consciousness in a state of bliss is the closest in existence to the state of absolute existence. In the final state all individuality is lost, and only the pure absolute remains. It is the stage when even bliss seems inadequate and a poor, unnecessary diversion and the Advaitist seeks to merge with this unqualified absolute. It is the state of perfect freedom because we have no more desires. It is the stage when we are everything, when there is nothing beyond us and nothing disturbs us. In this stage of total calmness, there is nothing more to be known or sought after. The ultimate purpose of life in Hinduism is to achieve this state of complete freedom. True religion in India means knowing the absolute in this way, and all spiritual efforts are only a preparation for this end.

The next question that arises is, how are we sure that the experience of mysticism is a true experience and not a delusional one? We know that drunks and mad men have delusions of fear, anger, and so on. How do we know that the mystical experience of oneness is not a similar delusion, only a positive one this time? How do we know that the paths of Yoga do not somehow produce a reaction in the mind, so that the mystical experience is simply a trick of the brain brought about in abnormal circumstances?

The experience of the mystical state, the sense of bliss, is sometimes mimicked by various other experiences such as drugs, fasting, asphyxiation, and physical ordeals such as high fever and torture. This seems to show that mystical experiences also are only a quirk of the brain, and not any experience of a higher truth. Can mystical experience be a spiritual goal when not only spirituality, but also all these other causes can give us similar experiences?

The answer really lies in what we consider ourselves to be— whether we consider our individual consciousness to be a stand-alone entity or having Brahman at its root. It really depends on our philosophical position with regard to consciousness. If we accept that there is an absolute consciousness at the base of our individual consciousness, then we are led by logic to accept that once our individual consciousness dies out, the absolute alone will remain, and hence mystical experience is the experience of this absolute field. But if we do not accept such an entity, then there can be no true mysticism and mystical experience can be seen to be nothing more than any other state of the mind.

We will know the ultimate truth only when we are finally able to scientifically discover the mystery of consciousness and of existence in general, and whether the Advaitic explanation is the true one. At present, the final question, whether there is an absolute beyond this world or not, can only be answered through logic and rational arguments. Accepting the mystical experience as true would depend on whether we accept the Advaitic philosophy or not. Once we accept the Advaitic metaphysical explanation of the world, we would be required to accept the mystical experience also as a true one when we follow its deductions to their logical end.

A close understanding of the Advaitic explanation for mysticism shows us that these experiences with drugs and so forth can be explained within the Advaitic position. In Advaita the state of mystical experience, or samadhi, is also a natural state, which is not discontinuous from the other states of our consciousness. It is not something that comes from outside, it is not a state that our consciousness changes into; rather, it is a state of consciousness itself and is continuous with our other states such as dreamless sleep, dreams, and the waking state. It is the purest state of our consciousness, and all other states are merely a derivation from it.

In fact, all the states of our individual consciousness may be considered to be a mystical experience. The difference is only in how far they are from the absolute state of consciousness. The differentiation from this pure state is brought about by our thoughts and feelings—that is, by the brain itself, which produces these thoughts. Once this differentiation is suppressed by any means, we regain what is already potential in us. Hence we may say that the experience of samadhi is not fundamentally different from these other experiences of our mind. This is the supreme naturalism of the Advaita, which rejects all non-natural causes of the world, including the mystical experience.

Based on such an understanding of the mystical experience, we can account for the experiences of drugs and so on. Drugs have always been used to duplicate the mystical experience since time immemorial. The most common drug is alcohol, which has been known since the Vedic ages, when the juice of a plant called *soma* was much extolled. Another famous drug in India is *bhang*, or marijuana. It is particularly connected to Shiva worship and is a constant accessory for the ascetics of India. In modern times, drugs like LSD and other hallucinatory substances are claimed from time to time to give a mystical experience.

The effect of all these agents can be understood as the decreasing of the control of thoughts on our awareness. They cause a state of passivity in the brain, much like sleep, and decrease its thought content. Our thoughts, feelings, and so forth are modulated by our brain activity, and hence it is perfectly possible that a modulation in a particular way of the physical and chemical states of the brain will lead to a change in the state of our thoughts and feelings. Once we accept that the Brahman consciousness lies at the base of our individual consciousness, we can logically accept that any state that leads to a weakening of our thoughts and awareness could also give an experience similar to samadhi.

So the effect of drugs can be seen to simply lead to a decrease in the thought-sensations content of the brain, a decrease in its ripples, in much the same way as Yoga. But Advaita rejects these practices because they give a false view of the same truth and do not lead to realization. The samadhi brought about in Yoga is not of a fundamentally different nature than the state brought about through drugs, but it differs in the *quality* of the mental state that it reaches.

These other experiences, such as drug use, do not reach that pure freedom but instead give only a distorted view of that supreme experience. These practices do not give true samadhi, because rather than controlling our thoughts, they deform them, and hence they are considered to be *tamasic*. The experiences that they bring about are not those of samadhi but are only mimics. In Yogic samadhi, the mind becomes pure and tranquil, and because of this tranquility the true nature of our individuality manifests itself.

But in such alternate practices, the mind is subdued by forces outside it and becomes weak, and this may at times lead to experiences that duplicate mysticism. But instead of the freedom that the mind attains in samadhi, here the mind is further trapped in by forces outside its control. Hence such experiences cannot give us the true freedom experienced in samadhi and do not lead to any meaningful insight or wisdom. Rather than strengthening us, they make us weak and powerless.

However, these experiences are still important in one way, because they show us that the mystical experience is in fact possible and is not just a myth. These distorted visions only serve to show the strength and power that can be received from a true mystical experience. Advaita, it must be remembered, is a search for truth, not a search for a God. It does not reject any practice that would give us the experience of the absolute. But these "shortcuts," on close examination, do not lead us to a true mystical experience; instead they lead us away from the path, weakening and eventually destroying us.

The harmful physical effects of drugs through addiction and ill health are already known. Other things like asphyxiation and high fever also act in a similar way, but all cause, or are the effects of, physical weakness. These acts are able to give us their effects only because they sort of bludgeon our minds into passivity, and hence they are inevitably harmful to us and lead to a weakening of body and mind.

But Yoga depends on a strong body and mind, and the exercises of Hatha Yoga were developed to ensure this. The highest state, *Sattva*, arising from a position of strength, and the lowest state, *Tamas*, arising from a position of weakness, always seem superficially similar. One arises from a mind that is in total control, and the other from a mind that is under suppression. In the same way, the mystical experience and drug intoxication, although seeming to be comparable at first, are in fact radically different both in their causes and their effects.

> *I do not know whether I was then a man*
> *dreaming I was a butterfly,*
> *Or whether I am now a butterfly*
> *dreaming I am a man.*

—Chuang Tzu, Zen philosopher

The question of death, too, is intimately related to our understanding of mysticism. Is death the final end to us, or can we hope to continue to exist in some other, more final form?

The answer to this also depends on whether we consider ourselves to be the individual self or the infinite Brahman. There certainly seems to be no possibility of the individual self surviving after death. Our self is bounded up in our memories, thoughts, and emotions generated in the brain's neurological circuits. There is no way in which they could survive the dissolution at death. On the other hand, if we are the infinite Brahman and the individual self, and our ego was only a contraction, then death would in fact be a release from this limitation, and we would experience a tremendous freedom at death.

Our relative consciousness and our individual ego and thoughts, feelings, and so on are a limited form of Brahman and have Brahman as their basis. So our true individuality is the individuality of Brahman, limited by our thoughts and feelings. So when our thoughts and feelings die out, our sense of individuality will not die out but will expand, and will be one with the absolute Brahman. At this stage, as in the final stage of samadhi, we will not have our individual self anymore but only the absolute self.

Hence if we consider ourselves to be the individual ego, then death is certainly final for us. But if we see ourselves as the infinite Brahman and this individuality as only a contraction, then death is not an end but an expansion. Again, Brahman is not an inert field, but it must have the property of absolute consciousness, as the relative consciousness is manifested from it. When our consciousness expands into the universal consciousness of Brahman, it does not cease to exist but exists on a plane that is immeasurably vaster than this, the plane of the absolute. Of course, there is no way to understand what such an existence would mean, because we can only understand living in an individual ego. But the accounts of mystical experiences certainly give us an immense hope of something immeasurably beautiful and great, something that cannot fail to fill us with hope and wonder.

In most of the interpretations of the Upanishads, such a definition of death, where the individual self attains the freedom of the absolute, is promised only for the realized souls, who during their lives have raised their self-awareness to such a height that only the faintest connection tied them down to their ego. But in many other passages, there is no such rider and death is seen as the final samadhi for all.

Perhaps the near-death experiences related by many people are an indication of this reality. They apparently indicate the individual consciousness expanding into the absolute as a result of the brain slowly dying, and perhaps indicate the experience that we will all undergo upon death. There are certainly many controversies surrounding such accounts, including the serious objection that many accounts give varying descriptions, and at least a few appear to be fake. But still, they do give hope that death is not a simple blankness but an expansion into the vastness of the infinite.

Perhaps, ultimately, such things will be known by scientific investigation. Science is the investigation of the external world, whereas mysticism is an investigation of the internal one. Scientific methods are more certain because they have the advantage of objectivity, in that they can be duplicated and observed by others. Mystical experiences, on the other hand, are subjective by their very nature.

It is of course vital to understand what consciousness is before we can try to understand mysticism. With the progress of science, we are probing deeper and deeper into understanding consciousness. It is only when we finally understand consciousness that we will be able to prove or disprove the Advaitic view that the absolute is the basis for our consciousness and, through this understanding, comprehend the mystical experience as well.

Different Paths to Mysticism

The absolute can be known not through one method only but by following many different ones. The four main methods set out in Hinduism are Jnana Yoga, Raja Yoga, Bhakti Yoga, and Karma Yoga. Besides these, there are many other paths, such as Tantricism and ascetic practices. But as Vivekananda pointed out, this did not mean that the four paths were exclusive to one another. Instead, he gave the analogy of the bird, whose head was Jnana Yoga, the two wings Bhakti and Karma, and Raja the tail. For the bird to fly, all these parts are equally necessary, and so also the Yogi must follow the precepts of all Yogas. But depending on their temperament, they may emphasize the practice that is most suitable for them.

The absolute can be understood in many different aspects: as something to be known or realized, as something to be loved, as something to be united with through strength of will, and as something to be united with through tranquility. Seeing it as something to be known, the Jnana Yogi asks the central question of the Mundaka Upanishad, "What is that knowledge, by knowing which, all this can be known?" Taking it as something to be loved, the Bhakta asks, "what is that love, by having which all this love can be known?" The Raja Yogi again seeks to know infinite power, and the Karma Yogi infinite peace.

The basic aim of all these paths is to achieve one-pointedness of mind—that is, to make the thoughts concentrated so that only one thought remains, until even that becomes finer and finer before ultimately disappearing.

In Jnana Yoga, this is done by analyzing a particular thing then examining and rejecting each thought that comes about it, until one reaches the essence of that thing. In Bhakti, it is done by filling the mind with love for the ideal, until only the thought of love remains in the mind. In Karma, this is achieved through cultivating detachment from all tasks, so that our thoughts, which are associated with our daily life, die down. In Raja Yoga, it is done by conscious concentration on any particular object until the mind becomes filled with that object only.

Mystics in other religions like Christianity and Islam also described their paths in detail, and rich traditions of mysticism developed in all religions of the world. But in these religions, the path described was mainly the path of love and devotion, the *Bhakti Yoga* of Hinduism. We also find some descriptions of practices that are reminiscent of other forms of Yoga, such as some of the breathing exercises and "navel gazing" of Christianity and the dervishes in Islam. But it is only in Hinduism that we find so many diverse paths to the mystical experience, allowing us a much wider variety of methods to choose to follow.

In Hinduism not just the paths of Yoga but all paths, including the arts, can lead to a mystical experience. Arts like music and dance also have mysticism as their goal. The goal here is to immerse oneself in the music to such an extent that all things but the music are forgotten and the mind becomes focused. In the Indian *ragas*, for example, the singer concentrates on a particular aspect of the music so that both he or she and the listener are led deeper and deeper into it, and nothing else is felt. The mind then becomes focused, and both the singer and the listener become so immersed in the song that ultimately even the song is left behind and samadhi is experienced. This is the goal of Indian classical music. In this way all other arts, such as dance, literature, and painting, also lead the way to mysticism.

Mysticism is enjoying a resurgence throughout the world. People everywhere are rediscovering the mystical traditions of their ancestors and that of others in the world, and using them for their spiritual quest. Perhaps this signifies a new age, where there will once again be a search into our internal world, and a desire to understand it, along with the desire to explore the external world. True religion such as this will be free from all political and social evils. It will not act as a divisive force, but will instead spread happiness throughout the world, both for the individual and for the whole of humanity.

10

Bhakti Yoga

You are the Gods of wind,
  Death, fire and water;
The moon; the Lord of life;
  and the great Ancestor.
I pay homage to You, O Lord,
  I pay homage a thousand times.

—**Bhagavad Gita, 11.39**

Bhakti Yoga is the path in which union with God is achieved through faith in a personal god. *Bhakti* is usually translated as devotion or worship, but in the Hindu sense it means more than just that. Bhakti means a complete emotional and spiritual immersion in the *love* for God. As the great Bengali saint Ramakrishna Paramahamsa said, "It begins in love, is continued in love and ends in love of God."

In its first stages of development in human religion, the path of worship began with deification of the forces of nature that confronted our ancestors. The first conceptions of divinity they formed were therefore of beings who were often more cruel than kind; beings that ruled over all the violence our ancestors faced. In the Rig Veda, the earliest hymns contain gods such as Indra and Rudra: gods who are at once violent and kingly, who hold power over humanity. The hymns try to win their favor through prayers, praise, and the offering of cattle and other gifts. There are numerous other gods who must be placated because of their control over different aspects of nature. In fact, a passage in the Rig Veda describing the number of gods works out to the famous figure of thirty-three *crore*, or 330 million.

In Hinduism, this tradition of worship of gods of nature continues to the present day. The number of gods to be worshipped and their respective powers present a bewildering array. There is the goddess Sitala Mata, for example, who holds power over smallpox and can keep it at bay. That at least seems to be one godhead that modern science has annihilated! Each village has its own deities, peaceful or malevolent, lurking about large trees and ponds, and these are regularly propitiated either out of superstitious fear or habit. However this worship, the persistence of the most primitive form of religion, is not what is meant by Bhakti.

Hinduism has another form of worship that is more universal and has a more discriminating tradition behind it. It is the worship of gods who hold special power over certain aspects of social life. Most of these gods and goddesses are derived from the Puranas and can be traced back ultimately to the Vedas. The Puranic world is one of rich imagery, myths, and symbols and is an inexhaustible saga of thousands of heavenly deities. Many of the tales are allegorical, but quite a few appear to have little more behind them than lively, child-like fantasy. The myths can have several layers of meaning, from simple tales of chivalry, faith, lust, and all other human virtues and failings, to a profound message of illumination.

These tales also have humans in them, including sages who have their own adventures, often threatening the gods themselves. Tales also include the Asuras, the dark forces pitted against the gods who are depicted as not only savage and cruel, but also as extremely strong, though they are always defeated in the end. There is often a hint of sympathy in the scriptures for these underdogs, who are sometimes defeated by the gods only by subterfuge. The tales can also turn out to be contradictory, so that a god who appeared as brave and dashing in one tale might turn out to be a coward in another. Thus, in the Puranas, Indra (the warrior of the Vedas) becomes one of the assembly of gods and loses much of his stature, being defeated by the Asuras, and on one occasion hiding in a lotus stalk to evade them.

In the course of time, individual gods came to acquire special powers over different aspects of human social life such as knowledge, wealth, and craftsmanship, and are identified through these powers. Every field of human endeavor came to have its own god as its presiding deity. As a god became more and more powerful, litanies devoted to him or her were composed, and particular days were fixed for their worship. These litanies would define the way of worshipping the god, the myths relating to the god, and his or her powers. They also described various features of the god, including some important points such as how many arms the God had and what each one of them held, and also their vehicles, which ranged from elephants to rats. The use of animals as vehicles gave sanctity to that animal in society. The goddess of learning, Saraswati, has a swan for her vehicle, and it is said that each swan will have a day in its life when the goddess will ride on its back. Because of this, it is considered lucky to keep swans around the house.

Particular professions usually have their own favorite relevant gods, and there is also a wide regional difference in the popularity of different gods. Besides Saraswati there is Lakshmi, the goddess of wealth, and Ganesha, who is worshipped for success in endeavors and hence is much in demand in the business community. There is the god Vishwakarma, who is the god of machinery, an engineer, and an architect rolled into one. He has been well-adapted into the modern age, and it is quite common to see Hindus offering incense and worship in front of various machines, such as motorcars and computers, on the day of his worship. Various manifestations of the gods are also worshipped. There is one story of Krishna who appeared as half-man and half-woman in a certain myth. This form is worshipped by the eunuch community in India, whose members are known as *hijras* and live in a separate, very tightly knit society.

Unlike the tree, pond, and disease spirits, the worship of such gods has religious and orthodox sanction. There is hardly a Hindu who will not worship a particular god at least on his or her special day. The worship of these gods, with their strange forms and characteristics, might seem incongruous at first sight and has often been under attack by reformers who see them as ancient superstitions. But on closer look, we find that it is not really so primitive after all.

Practically every aspect of Hinduism is imbued with religion in one way or another. There is hardly anything in Hindu life that is secular. There are vital religious ceremonies to go through during birth, death, and marriage, with important rituals for such things as the weaning day of the baby, menarche, and so forth. All Indian arts are also, in a sense, a spiritual striving. Indian classical dances like the Bharat Natyam have a deep religious core, and the goal of the dancer is to try to invoke the deity with his or her dance. Similarly, in Indian classical music, which is perhaps the oldest form of music extant today, the music is seen as a path to mystical experience. The Lord is experienced within oneself at the height of the song by both the singer and the listener.

Indians are proud of saying that they have at least one festival for each day of the year, and nearly all these festivals, excepting the spring festivals like the Bihu of Assam, are religious festivals. Behind the ornate customs and rites that mark each event in a Hindu's life, we find this core of spirituality trying to invoke something that is of a higher nature than this world.

The real significance of these deities lies in this attempt in Hinduism to spiritualize every aspect of life. We all strive for perfection in our efforts in any direction, whether in pursuit of knowledge, skill, or, more mundanely, wealth or success. This ideal of perfection is what is personified in the form of a deity in Hinduism and worshipped. It is an attempt to lend a spiritual dimension to the quest for perfection in that field. To achieve this personification of the ideal, a complex metaphor has to build up that will contain all the various aspects of perfection.

This explains the metaphor of the image, which is more like a visual metaphor of an ideal and is symbolic in nature. The forms of the deities, the numerous arms with their objects and their vehicles, are all symbols of different powers of the gods. They are considered necessary for perfection in that field. The whole form is supported by the myths built up around it and extolled in the hymns written in highly evocative Sanskrit using sophisticated language and imagery. The worshippers take the help of the image and the worship not as an end in itself but so that they can feel this ideal of perfection in themselves. This search for perfection in an imperfect world makes our worldly efforts into a spiritual quest. It is this spirituality that is sought by the worshippers as they bow before the image.

But even this is not Bhakti. For the goal of Bhakti is mystical, to experience the divinity within one's own self. The Bhakta seeks only to love, and, through this love, to touch the Lord. Pure love and merging with God through love is the aim of Bhakti.

The path of Bhakti begins in the earliest scriptures of India, the Vedas. It is here that we find, behind the simple nature worship of many hymns, the first steps of Bhakti. But it was in the scriptures of the later Gangetic civilization that Bhakti Yoga was truly developed as a philosophy. The great epics of India, the Ramayana and the Mahabharata, were composed here, along with the Puranas and the Agamas, including the Tantric texts. These scriptures yielded the gods of the three main channels of Bhakti in Hinduism: *Vaishnavism*, *Shaivism*, and *Tantricism*, the worship of the Mother Goddess. The main panegyric texts for the gods were also composed here: the Bhagavat Puran for Vishnu, and the Agamas for Shiva and the Mother Goddess. Several technical and explanatory texts relating to Bhakti are also from this period.

Bhakti Yoga continued to be developed and studied in several places in the country through the centuries. The texts relating to this philosophy are interesting in that they treat the subject as a science and detail the various stages of the aspirants in the path of Bhakti without a mysterious air. They are more like psychological studies, and the often extraordinary reactions of the aspirants and the dangers they face are described systematically and in a matter-of-fact manner. They were used carefully as guides by other Bhaktas, who would in turn add their own knowledge, and so Bhakti gradually acquired a considerable body of literature.

Another important development in the last millennium was the spread of Bhakti as a social movement. From being an individual method of worship, Bhakti took on a collective aspect. The commentaries of the dualistic Madhava and that of Ramanuja around the tenth century CE gave a fresh impetus to its growth. The advent of Islam also played an important part, both by posing a challenge to Hinduism and through the message of Sufism.

A number of teachers, including Chaitanya Mahaprabhu and Kabir, organized a social movement and began spreading the message of Bhakti. Their followers formed sects and spread their message of love and inclusion. The Bhaktas declared their call for equality and opened the doors of divine experience to all. It worked as a form of revolt against the class and caste combination of society, thereby weakening its grip. It was vital in preserving Hinduism against first the spread of Islam, and later Christianity.

Another such important teacher was Sankardeva in Assam, around the fifteenth century CE. Before Sankardeva, Assam was in the grip of the Tantric cult, which by then had become degraded. Magic and superstition filled the land, and religion was more like a sword hanging over one's head than a means to spirituality. It was at this time that Sankardeva began to spread his message of *ekasaran*, devotion to a single god, and advocated Bhakti as the only path to reach God. This was vital in rejuvenating the Assamese society, and Assam became an important stronghold of Bhakti.

Bhakti begins with an ideal: the loved one. This is the concept of the personal god: a god who has "personal" involvement with us, who is moved by our prayers and our plight, who has power over our lives. Such a god is conceived as one who loves us, who rules over us, and who guides us at every turn.

All over the world, in every society, this concept of a personal god has risen independently, though with different attributes. Humanity has always felt in its heart the touch of such a being, which is the perfection of all the ideals we most aspire to, such as love, beauty, and truth. By necessity, humans have conceived of God in terms of a human appearance. In terms of gender, most religions with a single god conceive it as male. In Hinduism, though, with its multiple deities, there are both male and female gods, and in some traditions such as the Tantric, the presiding deity is female. Sometimes the personal god is thought of as formless, like Allah in Islam, but even then, his or her actions are conceived in human terms.

In contrast to impersonal conceptions, a personal god is aware and affected by human actions and also interacts with us, whether in responding to our prayers, loving us, or in sitting in judgment over us. The conception of a personal god defines God as an all-powerful and all-knowing being. As Swami Vivekananda said, "He is the Eternal, the Pure, the Ever-Free, the All-Knowing, the All-Merciful, the Teacher of all teachers."

The ideal of a personal god in Hinduism is called *Ishwar*. In Hinduism, there is no single word like "God" that wraps up all our conceptions; instead there are different words for different conceptions, from the impersonal to the personal. Ishwar delineates the personal god.

In Bhakti, Ishwar is always defined as loving. Love is the very essence of the Hindu conception of God and his way of relating to us. He does not sit in judgment over us, punishing us for our sins or rewarding us for good, nor is there any talk of hell in relation to Ishwar. "He, the Lord is, of his own nature, inexpressible love." Ishwar is a sea of love, and we have only to open our hearts to let that sea flow in and fill us.

Although the concept of a personal god prevails in virtually all cultures throughout the world, there is a great deal of difference in the way in which such a god is defined. Vivekananda marked out the three ways in which God is understood in various systems. These are the ways of the dualist, the qualified monist, and the monist. The difference, of course, arises from the difference in how the nature of the universe is perceived in the system—that is, the metaphysics of the religion. But although the interpretation of Ishwar is different, the goal of Bhakti in all three systems is essentially the same, as it is in all of Hinduism. The aim is to experience the truth within oneself, and to experience union with God. This goal of mysticism is common to all religions.

The first is the way of the pure dualists. For them there is a clear distinction between the Lord and the universe. The Lord stands alone, away from the universe. It is he who has created this universe and who rules over us, supporting and sustaining us. The dualists see Ishwar as outside themselves, as a separate existence to whom they offer themselves. The individual soul, the *jiva*, is thus completely separate from Ishwar. Madhava, the dualist commentator, is emphatic in defining the distinction between Ishwar and jiva, the individual soul. The jiva, by its very nature, is limited and can never have the unlimited power of Ishwar. The only way is to pray and worship Ishwar so that he may take the soul into his shelter and relieve it forever from the cycle of rebirth to which it is doomed.

The next is the way of the qualified monists. For them, Ishwar is the core from which all individual souls have sprung, like the flame and sparks. Ishwar is the soul of the universe in the same way as the jiva is the soul of the body. They believe that the human soul is a part of God, and hence God lies within all of us. The qualified monists believe in a personal god, a god who wills and who creates the world as a spider spins out the silk from its own body. Ishwar is the whole, and the soul is a part. So though the world is created both by and from God, there is always a difference between the world and God. Hence there is always a difference between the individual soul and God, the difference of part and whole.

The final step is that of the monism of Advaita. Advaita recognizes only one absolute truth, the truth of Brahman. Brahman, the absolute principle, is the only existence, and all others are illusionary, as they have only relative existence. Brahman, by its very nature, is impersonal; there is no question of it being affected by human predicaments. This Brahman, an existent principle, cannot really be called "God" in the sense that we normally understand by the term, which usually suggests a personal being. But as this Brahman is the end of Advaitic religious efforts, it may be referred to as "God" in a broader sense of the term.

For the Advaitist, it is the absolute, seen through the mind, which is seen as Ishwar. Ishwar is the highest reading of the absolute by the mind. The mind cannot of itself conceive of the absolute, hence it must conceive of it as a being with attributes. Since such attributes belong to the Brahman, they are considered to be perfect, and this is the Ishwar of the Advaitist.

In this sense, for the Advaitists, Bhakti is a vital aid to achieve the truth. Meditation on the impersonal Brahman, the absolute, is very difficult. The mind needs something, a point, to concentrate on. By concentrating on the personal god through Bhakti, the Advaitists are able to develop their concentration to the point that they achieve merger with the personal god. They then go further and strike down even the personal god, to achieve final samadhi with the impersonal absolute. Through this, Bhakti makes the way easier for the aspirants of Advaitism.

It may seem at first that Bhakti does not conform to Advaita, and so an Advaitist could never have true Bhakti. Bhakti demands a personal god to love, and the truth by definition in Advaita is far beyond both personal and impersonal. Advaita, being a single-minded intellectual pursuit of the truth, has no use for such criticism and is ready to use whatever it feels is needed to achieve its goal. If Bhakti makes the way easier, then it cannot be neglected.

But it is not just this cold-blooded sense of purpose that drives advaitic teachers. The capacity for spiritual love is infinite in humans, and we find in many advaitic writers a description of Bhakti that is as emotional and profound as in any dualistic teaching. The saint Shankaracharya himself was a great Shiva Bhakta and composed many exquisite hymns of devotion. He also established four important *peeths* of Shiva worship in the four corners of India, which are still important centers of learning for Advaita.

The main reason that Bhakti is considered important for the Advaitist is that this path of Yoga uses the faculty of love. Love is considered to be the most intense force available to the human mind. By using this force through Bhakti, the Yogi is able to tap a vital power of his mind. Strict Jnana or Raja Yogis who do not accept a personal god are not able to make use of this strength in their struggle. The knowledge obtained through pure Jnana Yoga is said to make the Yogi a dry and hard man. Only a strict ascetic can pursue this harsh path, and madness always lies in the fringes. Hence Vivekananda preached that Yogis should practice all four paths of Yoga, putting the maximum emphasis on the path to which they have a natural inclination.

Advaita gives a basis for understanding the difference in conceptions of the personal god in different philosophies. The Advaitist says that, in fact, it is the idea of the Advaita that lies beyond all Bhakti texts and in all devotional philosophies everywhere. The three ways in which God is understood are considered the three stages through which the aspirant passes in Bhakti, with the Advaitic stage being the ultimate stage. All Bhakti movements are considered by Advaitists to have as their inmost teaching that of non-dualism, the dualist and qualified monist being only the initial stages for the aspirant. These stages are taught initially to the aspirants, as the last stage of Advaitic Bhakti may be difficult to grasp at first; the teachers of Bhakti thus lead the aspirant up gradually. All such paths are believed to end ultimately in the non-dualistic conception. The dualistic and qualified monistic interpretations are not regarded as incorrect, but as steps on the way to Advaita, the highest teaching.

Such threefold teaching can be discerned quite clearly in the teaching of Chaitanya Mahaprabhu and other teachers of the Bhakti movement. This teaching is also found in the theology of Sankarveda of Assam, who preached the principle of *matibheda*, or the difference in the mental capacity of the disciples, and accordingly taught different ways to the disciples, with Advaitic Bhakti being reserved for the innermost circle.

According to Advaitists, these three stages of Bhakti are also found in religions outside India. In Christianity too, the three different interpretations of God and mysticism can be traced. The goal of mysticism, to experience the divine within oneself, was sought solely through the path of devotion in Christianity. The use of any other way such as the meditation of Raja Yoga or the discrimination of Jnana Yoga would contradict essential church doctrines. Most teachers also accepted that Christianity was the only way, with Christ as the only mediator. There was never anything like the frequent Hindu teaching that one has to rise above religion itself. Also, unlike in Hinduism, where the mystical experience is the goal of all religion, in Christianity this idea was never widely accepted; the story of Christian mysticism is one of only a number of schools and teachers who practiced in isolation.

Yet it is remarkable how closely Christian mystical writings resemble that of Bhakti Yoga. Virtually all important ideas in Bhakti find their mirror in Christianity. The three strands of mysticism—dualistic, qualified monistic, and the pure non-dualistic—are clearly visible in different schools.

Mysticism in Christianity starts with Christ, who taught his own perfect union with his Father. The Bible frequently refers to mystical goals, "blessed are the pure in heart, for they shall see God," (Matthew 5:8). This was found most clearly in the letters of Paul and the gospel according to John.

The dualistic mysticism is the most common path and is also recognized by the official church, to some extent. For most of Christianity, it was not a merger with God but "seeing" God, an essentially dualistic doctrine. "Each of these," wrote the medieval Dutch mystic, Jan van Ruysbroeck, "keeps its own nature." Here God and man are two different substances, and even when man sees God, the two remain separate. This strand of mysticism is seen most clearly in Catholics and the Eastern Church.

Again, many mystics taught a form of qualified monism. They preached, like William Law, the English spiritual writer and mystic, that "that the eternal Word of God lies hid in thee, as a spark of the divine nature." Seeing God thus becomes a merger in one's inmost being. With qualified monism, one experiences God within oneself and feels oneself to be divine. Mystics such as St.Teresa declared, "It is plain enough what unity is—two distinct things becoming one." One thus merges with Jesus himself.

Some mystics went beyond this and introduced a concept that was as monistic as that of Brahman. One of the earliest writers was Dionysus the Areopagite, who distinguished "the super-essential Godhead" from all positive terms ascribed to God, the "not this, not this" of Advaita. Meister Eckhart declared that the soul of man and the Son of God were one, "let us pray to God that we may be free of God." This radical form of Christian mysticism emphasized the absolute unknowability of God. They suggested that true contact with the transcendent involves going beyond all that we speak of as God—even the Trinity—to an inner "God beyond God," a divine darkness or desert in which all distinction is lost.

In Islam also, we find the tradition of mysticism, mainly in the Sufi tradition. From the earliest days, mysticism was an important part of the Islam religion. The mystics drew from the Qu'ran for their teachings. Although the Qu'ran preached a formless God, it spoke also of the love of God and the love of his followers for him. This was used as the base for the philosophy of Sufism.

As in Christianity, however, mysticism never emerged as an integral movement but remained confined to isolated teachers and their followers. In Islam, several mystics arose who spoke out their intense love for God, and their nearness to him, in some of the most beautiful language ever created. As the various mystics spread their individual message, we find a number of different interpretations of the Sufi tradition. But behind these apparently confusing teachings, there is the same universal interpretation of God in three ways: the dualistic, the qualified monistic, and the monistic.

Rabi'ah al-'Adawiyah (died 801 CE), a woman from Basra (now Iraq), first formulated the Sufi ideal of a love of God that was disinterested, without hope for paradise and without fear of hell. In the hymns of the earliest mystics, we find expression of this love for God, where the mystics spoke of joining all nature in the praise of God. These ideas were derived from the Qu'ran and were purely dualistic.

Gradually, we find other ideas being developed. The union of being theory suggested that all existence is one, a manifestation of the underlying divine reality. Hallaj, one of the most well-known of the Sufis, declared that "God loved himself in his essence, and created Adam in his image." Thus the idea of qualified monism gradually gained ground. This was totally against the orthodoxy, which came out in full force in opposition, and Hallaj himself was executed. Such views could not be suppressed, however, and much of Sufism has, as its basis, what is understood in Hindu philosophy as qualified monism.

This idea was taken even further by some mystics, especially in India, perhaps under the influence of Hinduism, and a non-dualistic conception was developed. Here we find an emphasis on the idea of divine unity, which borders on becoming monism, and the distinctions between God and the world (and humans) tend to disappear. Official Islam and other mystics vigorously contested this idea, believing that it went too far. However, it had taken root in India, and even today it continues to have a strong influence on Islam.

Due to the difference in definitions, the teachings of Bhakti had varying views on the endpoint that would be attained by the aspirants. Because of the difference in the goals sought, there is a difference in the goals attained. Dualists seek only to see the Lord and to feel sheltered by the presence of the Lord. This is the goal achieved by their Bhakti. Qualified monists seek only to feel the Lord within themselves, to feel they are one with the Lord, and to merge with the personal Ishwar. They too achieve their goal.

But Advaitists seek the ultimate truth. They must go beyond the personal, beyond the impersonal, and achieve the final experience of merging with that beyond which there is nothing else, the absolute. They too achieve their goals with their Bhakti. Dualists see Ishwar as outside themselves and offer themselves to Ishwar. Qualified monists see themselves as a part of Ishwar, but only as a small and restricted part.

The vision of the Advaitists is different. They see no difference between Ishwar and themselves, as they themselves are Ishwar, "I am That, I am That." The dualistic and qualified monistic mystical experiences are only stages on the path to the final culmination in the Advaitic merging with God. The Advaitist says the dualist should not stop at dualism, nor should the qualified monist stop at his or her vision, but that they should go onward. They will then find that the God they sought outside themselves is to be found inside. If they go on further, they will come to the ultimate realization that there is no difference between the Lord and themselves—they themselves are God. At this stage all distinctions will dissolve, there will be no manifestation and no consciousness. Thus the aspirant achieves the final goal of Bhakti, merging in the absolute Brahman.

Having chosen the path of Bhakti, the aspirants must then choose a particular Ishta, or ideal, as their Ishwar. The personal god must take a form. There are numerous ideals throughout the world, and there have been probably more wars fought because of this multiplicity than for any other reason. Each culture has its own individual ideal, from Jesus, Allah, and Jehovah to other, lesser-known gods.

The unfolding of distinct ideals in each culture was inevitable. They are rooted in the land, language, and history of the community in which they evolved. Each carries the genius of that society and is the result of that society's cumulative experience. The history of a society gives it a unique outlook on life, and hence on its ideals. Thus every ideal is important, and it makes no sense to criticize or to make comparisons with others. Individuals also have their own way of understanding the chosen ideal, and provisions must be made for individual predilections.

The ideal may or may not have form, as that of Allah. Each such Ishta has its own myths and history behind it and its own particular form of worship. These ideals have evolved in a way that makes them powerful symbols, entrancing and drawing us onwards. There are the heroic tales of sacrifice for humanity, of wisdom, and, above all else, love. Love is the quality that characterizes all ideas of God irrespective of the culture of origin. Behind myths like creation and judgment days, the one universal idea is of this love. It is this aspect of our God that we must realize and fasten on to.

In the matter of choosing our particular ideal, we must all be guided from the heart. The form must be such that it inspires us and draws us onward. In general, the ideal of our upbringing is usually the most attractive for us. Among Hindus, each family and community usually follows a particular Ishta, and hence the child is drawn to it. Similarly, the ideal of Jesus for Christians and Allah for Muslims is already upheld for them and is the easiest for them to adopt.

One aspect of Hinduism that has always puzzled outsiders and led to suggestions that Hinduism is not a single religion is Hinduism's numerous Ishwars, or gods. The myths of the Puranas have yielded a huge number of deities, but in general, they can all be traced to three sources: Vishnu, Shiva, and the Mother Goddess. Vishnu is not worshipped as such but in the various forms of his avatars or incarnations, mainly Krishna and Ram. Krishna also has numerous avatars who are worshipped in different regions and temples.

The Mother Goddess, Shakti, is also worshipped in a bewildering number of forms, with practically each temple having a particular form, the most well-known of which are Kali, Durga, and

Kamakhya. Such is the variety of ideals that, as Vivekananda said, members within the same family could have different ideals. But in general, an individual's chosen ideal is usually that of a particular region, community, or caste.

This multiplicity of ideals in Hinduism is in sharp contrast to monotheistic religions like Christianity and Islam. But the basic truth is the same: the ideal of a personal god. As Ramakrishna Paramahamsa used to say, "From the same tank, the Hindu draws water and calls it *jal*, the Muslim calls it *paani*, and the Christian water, but the substance is the same." The Rig Veda declared thousands of years ago that "there is but one truth, the wise call it by various names." This tolerance embedded in Hinduism draws it apart from all other religions.

Once we select our ideal, which is not a conscious process as such but an unconscious one, we must stick to that alone. *Eka nishtha*, or devotion to one ideal, is absolutely necessary, especially to a beginner. We do not have to wait for faith to enter our hearts or to establish an intellectual belief in God before beginning worship. Each person should begin immediately giving all his heart to any God whose idea he or she accepts.

Doubts will arise in our hearts, said Ramakrishna. Such doubts are bound to arise in each heart, whether that of the simple-minded believer or the Advaitist. In fact, simple dualistic beliefs are more likely to be challenged by doubts as the believers find their prayers not answered. The Advaitists, praying to an ideal rather than a flesh and blood God, do not pray for such goals. But they are likely to have intellectual doubts as to whether they can have Bhakti toward a personal god when, at the same time, they assert that the truth is beyond both personal and impersonal. Doubts may arise regarding questions about the deity, the efficacy of Bhakti in respect to the absolute, and also regarding the superiority of Bhakti over Jnana Yoga and so forth.

The answer to such doubts is to continue with the practice. Yogis, once they have fixed their minds on following the path of Bhakti and have chosen their Ishta, cannot turn back and start arguing again. They must ignore doubts when they arise and not try to grapple with them, which would lead to wasted energy. The Upanishads assert that they have only to continue with their practice, and all their doubts will be solved and fall away. As long as the aspirants persist in their struggle, the answers will come by themselves when the time is ripe. The analogy given is that of a road up a hill: even though the road may be winding, and at times descending rather than climbing, by continuing along the road, we can be sure of reaching the top. As aspirants continue in their Bhakti, in time their faith becomes impregnable and doubts become more and more faint. But all doubts will finally be removed only when samadhi is attained, and the Yogi becomes one with the truth.

Once the path and the Ishta are chosen, we come to another important requisite in Hinduism: a guru. This aspect of Hinduism has always generated a great deal of controversy. The total faith that a guru demands often leaves the devotee open to exploitation, a fact that a horde of cheats have taken full advantage of. One must be especially careful in accepting a guru and remain always on guard. Like the other Yogas, Bhakti Yoga also has its technicalities that require explanation. Each aspirant will have their own individual problems, and it is only a teacher with enough experience who can provide the answers.

One advantage of Bhakti is that the schools of Bhakti are still extant and their knowledge is available in an unbroken tradition.

Many of the Bhakti teachers have established movements, which are still running today, centered around particular regions or temples. Each school has its own practices and teachings on the various nuances of Bhakti. Within these schools, the aspirants may find the direction they need.

Among these, the tradition of Ramakrishna Mission is one that still runs very strong. This is the school originally founded by Swami Vivekananda and the other twelve disciples of Ramakrishna, and it is a continuing and vibrant tradition. Another such important tradition, which has carried on in an uninterrupted line, is that of Sankardeva in the Assam province of India. It centers on institutions called *namghars* that Sankardeva established all over Assam, which are in fact growing stronger today. Other religions also have their own orders that can provide guidance for their followers. There are, for example, different churches and monasteries in Christianity, and the Sufi schools in Islam.

But all these traditional bodies are not immediately available to most of us. They usually demand much more time and effort than we can afford to give. However, even a little guidance is better than none, and even when we cannot spend much time, it is perhaps best if we keep some contact with such guides, however strenuous the process. When we are unable to do even this, books must be our guides.

But our ultimate guide must always be ourselves. If we have total faith, then we know that we can do no wrong in this path of love. Hence our true guru is *Satchidananda*, God himself.

The Preparation

As an ocean can be emptied by the tip of a blade of Kusa grass, so also can the mind be controlled by absence of unsteadiness.

—Mandukya Upanishad, III.42

The first step in the practice of Bhakti is *yama* and *niyama*, the dos and the don'ts. They consist of the cultivation of virtues like *satya*, *daya*, *ahimsa*, and *anabhidya*, and the control of passions like lust, greed, and anger. This is the ethical part of Bhakti. The goal of ethics here is the same as in other Yogas, to remove the "knots in the heart" and purify the Yogi for the struggle.

Satya means truth: speaking of things as they are. Daya means service to others. Service in Hinduism is meant to be done not just in a humanitarian sense but as an act of spirituality. Ramakrishna Paramahamsa advised that, while serving others, it must not be done with a sense of pity but rather with gratefulness that one has the chance to serve God. Ahimsa, or non-violence, is larger than simply not killing, it means not injuring others by word, deed, or even thought. Anabhidya means same-sightedness or tolerance, not discriminating against anyone.

The control of passions like lust, greed, and anger is advised in all paths of Yoga, as well as practically all religions. Controlling these most basic instincts is not an easy task for most of us, and such religious teachings end up making us feel inadequate in actual practice. The prospect of a life devoid of sensory pleasures also seems to lead to a rather unattractive and dreary sort of existence. Indeed, the very mention of having to give up lust is sure to scare away most people from taking up any path.

Other paths, such as Jnana, Raja, and Karma, assume that the aspirant does not have any of these passions and offers little help for anyone who has not controlled them, taking it as a sign of unfitness. All religions delight in simply commanding us to be free from them, often adding threats of an eternity in hell to add to the pressure.

But in Bhakti, we have the most natural way of conquering these feelings. For Bhakti does not insist on aspirants trying to control their urges forcefully, nor does it assume that they are free from these. It says that all passions and love of sense objects, that is, all desires, ultimately stem from our love for the divine. Our every thought, every desire, no matter how low it seems, has as its basis this desire of the soul for the absolute. The love for Brahman is manifested as the love for God, and the love for God is manifested as the love for the objects of our desires, due to our ignorance. It is the divine love for God that becomes corrupted into love for other sense objects.

We need not then fear our passions anymore, they are not monsters waiting to drag us into hell, nor like puritan philosophers need we think of them as expressions of our baseness. Instead, in Bhakti we realize that it is our desire to satisfy the inmost longing of our soul that leads us to such passions, and it is only our failure to understand them in their true light that makes us see some desires as low. There is thus no sin in Bhakti, or anything else to be ashamed of. Consciously or unconsciously, we are all striving for the same goal.

Once this idea is realized, the way to controlling our desires becomes clear. The yearning for God is our true nature, and all other desires are only offshoots from it. Hence, all we have to do is actively direct our minds to love for God, and all desires will become subsumed in this love. As our love for God grows stronger, our love for sense objects will become fainter accordingly. This is the simplest and most natural way of achieving control. We do not have to try to actively suppress our desires. Let the desires come as they will; we only need to persist with the love of God. Once the mind is turned toward the luster of God, the smaller objects will in time cease to have any attraction as they provide pleasure of much lesser quality. Hence we need not fret about giving up sex; Bhakti says we will do so automatically when we can access a bliss that is so much superior that sex ceases to attract us.

As long as this renunciation is not attained, however, the Bhaktas will have to live in the world surrounded by passions. They must then perform their actions like the Karma Yogi, by nonattachment to their actions. Unlike the narrow path of Karma Yoga, this too becomes much easier in Bhakti Yoga, for the Bhaktas can achieve this by simply doing their actions and then renouncing the fruits to the will of God. The devotees say that God will decide how and what fruit their action will bear. Thus they offer all actions to God and stop worrying about the fruits. This is the meaning of "thy will be done"—the Bhaktas cease to worry about actions and their results. They attain complete calmness and peace, and even while living in the world, achieve renunciation from it. This is much easier than trying to cultivate a rigid attitude of nonattachment to results, as in Karma Yoga.

Bhakti has many other guidelines for Yogis. One strict direction regards the company we keep. In Bhakti, more than in the other Yogas, this is important because it demands constant remembrance of God. Hence, we should try to remain in like-minded company as often as possible. This is another advantage of being part of a movement centered on Bhakti. Loose talk, by distracting our minds, will take us away from the path. We should try to arrange things in such a way that everything around us reminds us of God, like keeping pictures of God or other positive images in the house. (If someone says they look tacky, that's exactly the kind of company that we should be avoiding!) All things—such as music, books, and entertainment—should lead toward the divine, as far as possible.

In the cynicism of modern society, religion is often considered nonintellectual and superstitious. But it is false pride to say that one does not need this aspect of human emotion. The human mind is complex and difficult to understand and has several different aspects. The spiritual need is one of its most basic needs, whether we consider it to be a part of evolution or a God-given thing. One can ignore this only at the peril of not having one's character fully developed. Hence, all attempts to crush out religion, wherever they have been made, have failed. The need for spirituality is too great. One need not be ashamed of needing spirituality, just as no one would feel ashamed of saying that he or she yearns for good music or intellectual satisfaction.

A great deal of stress is also placed on food. Certain foods are believed In India to be exciting to the senses. These include, besides the obvious suspects like meat and alcohol, a long list of other foods, which seem quite innocuous, like onions and some pulses. All these foods are strictly avoided by orthodox Hindus. This became even more important in Bhakti, and great stress was laid on this point. This theory ultimately led to widespread vegetarianism in India.

Such strict observations can also have their drawbacks and lead to fanaticism, as among some Hindus when the upper castes refused to eat food on which even the shadow of an untouchable had fallen. Prominent teachers of Bhakti stressed that these rules are to be observed in moderation, and we should not forget that they are only accessories, not the true struggle.

Observing all these general rules of conduct are believed to lead to a cleansing of the mind and body of the aspirants. In this way, the aspirants feel themselves purified and become ready to follow the path of Bhakti Yoga.

The Ways and Means:

Meditating on the feet of Hara, O! we shall spend, in the holy forest, nights aglow with the beams of the full autumnal moon.

—Vairagya Satakam, 86

The aspirant in the path of Bhakti Yoga begins by observing all the outer rituals of worship. These rituals, when first performed, may seem meaningless, but one should remember that these ceremonies, myths, and worship of God are only links in a chain. There is no need to despise them. All the links lead up to the same center, and the Bhaktas need only to hold on to a link and draw themselves in. The one thing to remember is to keep going forward. In all these rituals, Bhakti teaches that there is an outer form and an inner form. Although rituals may at first be performed mechanically, the Bhaktas, as they go deeper and deeper, realize the inner meaning of these rituals, and perform them with greater understanding. Then, as they draw closer, the rituals are performed less and less until the final union is achieved, when all rituals are stopped. Bhakti begins with ritual worship and ends in union with the divine.

The dispute between observance of rituals and pure faith alone was characterized as the difference between the baby monkey and the kitten. The baby monkey holds on tightly to its mother as she moves about, while the kitten can only cry for its mother, which comes immediately and carries it about. Similarly, ritualists like the Purva Mimamsas laid emphasis on the observance of rituals to "cling" to God, whereas in Vedanta the accent is on having faith; deep faith by itself will bring God to the devotee. A similar dichotomy is also seen in Christianity between Catholicism, which believes in rituals, and Protestantism, which emphasizes faith that would bring salvation at God's discretion.

As is to be expected in a heterogeneous religion like Hinduism, the rituals of worship are of a diverse nature, and each region and sect has its own traditions. The Bhakti schools have their own rites of worship, and their respective followers follow these faithfully. The rituals are constantly modified in accordance with the changes in society. The bulk of Hindu rituals, however, are very ancient, and most rituals can be traced back (at least in seed form) to the Vedic age and even earlier. Hence we find in the rituals the simplicity of the nature worship of our first beginnings combined with the sophisticated theories of the highest philosophers.

The Bhakta in Hinduism begins by observing rituals like visiting temples, participating in the holy festivals, pilgrimages, the ritual worship of idols, singing of hymns, and finally prayer and meditation.

The worship of God through festivals is an important expression of the love of God. In Hinduism, God is not always worshipped with the grim reverence seen in other religions. Worshipping God can also be fun, and there are various festivals in India where the Lord is worshipped amid games and laughter. In the Rasa Leela, Krishna is worshipped in the attitude of enjoying himself on swings in the garden of Vrindavan. In Holi, the legend of Krishna sporting with the Gopis is celebrated with colors, while in Diwali, the cities light up for Ram's homecoming with lamps and crackers. The folk culture of India, its music, dances, and stories, are all celebrations, in one way or another, of some aspect of God.

Other religions have similar festivals, such as the Christmas and Easter of Christians and Eid of Islam. Hindus, though, can claim to have more of them than any other. As is perhaps inevitable, entertainment and commercialization have seeped into such festivals, but the core of spirituality is still strong in most people even as they take part in the celebrations, and in this way they help to bring fresh energy to the religion.

Going to holy places, like temples, is an important way of communicating with the divine. Churches, temples, and mosques serve the very important function of taking us into their own world, a world where the idea of God reigns supreme. They are embellished with intricate carvings, paintings, or other decorations in such a way as to create a spiritual atmosphere. They lead us away from the humdrum everyday world into a world that stands apart. This awakens a sense of enchantment and reminds us of the Spirit. We should use these temples to remind and refresh our spiritual quest. These temples and other holy places can be seen as important from a purely psychological viewpoint.

Another way of seeing this is that, over the ages, numerous holy persons have visited temples and other sacred places and millions of other devotees have left behind their prayers and yearning for God. It is believed in most religious traditions that thoughts have a sort of energy field. A combination of numerous such positive fields in the temples is believed to be purifying and leaves an imprint. While such a belief is not consistent with our present-day scientific knowledge, it is widely accepted in most religions, and adds to the atmosphere of piety.

Another reason is found in the architecture of the temples. Temple construction in India is done following strict guidelines, known as Vastu Shastra, regarding such things as the site, direction, walls, and so forth. Temples are built following a broad plan that mirrors the human body. Whereas the temple itself represents the body, the deity is usually found in a deeper enclosure beyond several doors, and represents the soul. This lies directly in the center of the temple and has a straight opening upward toward the sky, representing the upward path of the soul. The enclosure is usually dark and relatively small. The site of the temple is very important, and only sanctified spots as dictated by the *shastras* are selected. All this is believed to give the temple an intense spiritual field so that, as the devotee proceeds into the temple, he or she feels the actual presence of the divine and finds fulfillment of his or her Bhakti.

The importance of temples and other places of worship ultimately rests with the devotee. As long as they feed our inspiration, the temples can prove very useful in our quest.

Another important religious custom in Hinduism is the pilgrimage. Hinduism can lay claim to being the oldest religion in the world, and, over the centuries, certain places have become sanctified by customs and traditions as holy places. Among these, the foremost is the river Ganga, whose banks contain some of the most ancient cities in the world to be continually inhabited. These temple cities and their *ghats* (stairs leading down to the water) on the Ganga have drawn pilgrims since the dawn of civilization.

Some specific places, during certain conjunctions of stars as calculated by astrologers, are believed to be especially holy, such as the Kumbh Mela, and draw literally the highest congregation of humans at a single place. The Kumbh is so old that Huen Tsang, who witnessed it in the sixth century CE, described it even then as being the most ancient rite in the world. Temples all over the country are also important pilgrimage centers. Centuries of myths and traditions have given them such a great potency in the Hindu mind that a believer who is able to visit these places feels spiritually energized. Even if we consider it important only in a psychological sense, the pilgrimage remains a vital part of Hindu religious life.

The ritual worship of the Lord through his image is called *puja*. In Hinduism, this worship of God is done through nature. The produce of the earth—such as flowers, leaves, grass, natural fragrances, water from pure sources like holy rivers and lakes, and fire—are used in this worship. The gods have their own favorite flowers and other articles; for example, Krishna is worshipped with blue flowers and Shiva with bel leaves. Their use in worship has given a sense of holiness to several flowers and trees, such as the peepul tree, the lotus flower, and sandalwood. Use of milk and milk products like ghee and curds is mandatory, and the vessels used are of bronze, probably a throwback to the metal of the Indo-Saraswati civilization where it all began. The making of the idol itself is an intricate art and is performed by specialized sculptors. The idols are made of clay, stone, or metal, the most precious being a mixture of eight metals known as *asthadhatu*. The creation process for idols involves many rules and regulations regarding the form of the idol and specifying things such as the height-to-breadth ratio.

These idols are meant to be placed both in homes and in temples. Idol worship through puja is one of the most important features of Hinduism. The householder performs regular puja before the idols at specific times. In important temples, the image is treated as a king; elaborate rituals, patterned on the daily activities of a ruler, with the temple priests as his attendants, are performed. The image is woken up in the morning with hymns, then given a ceremonial bath and adorned, after which the morning puja is performed. The devotees are then allowed to pray before the image in the same way as a king holds an audience with his subjects. At noon, the king is offered his food, and only then can the others eat. The king then takes a noon siesta followed by a repeat audience for devotees and in the evening. There are even performances by temple dancers and singers in front of the image for entertainment. At night, the king and all his courtiers finally sleep. The older the temple, the more minutely are the rituals followed.

All this might seem at first to be idle superstition, but the important thing to recognize in these rituals is that it is not the idol that is worshipped but the God who is symbolized by the idol. As in all other traditions of Hinduism, it is the symbolism that is important, not the actual image. In fact, in religious festivals like Ganesh Chaturthi, Durga Puja, Saraswati Puja, and Vishwakarma Puja, the idol is made of clay, and after the days of worship, it is discarded in rivers or seas when the festival ends. The worship of idols can range from a simple fetishism to the highest achievement of spirituality. True Bhaktas understand this significance, and when they perform the rituals it is to the Lord and not the idol that they offer their puja. Ultimately, the symbolism becomes so potent that the presence of the Lord is experienced through the idol.

Another way the idol helps is during meditation, by giving the devotee a form to meditate on. The Yogic practices of meditation need an image to focus on, and the idol helps to provide this. Through the idol, the Yogi can visualize a form of the Lord and can thus meditate on that. Pujas also help by forming habits. When the Bhakta cultivates the daily puja, it becomes such a habit that by performing it, he is led into the mood of prayers and meditation. He can thus make a shift from the daily world into that of spiritualism. In this way, the ritual of the puja becomes an important part of meditation and prayers.

One of the most important and universal ways of worshipping the Lord is through the use of music with devotional hymns and songs. The appeal of music seems to be deeply ingrained into the human mind. Music has been used in all religions to communicate with the divine. In Hinduism, it found its earliest base in the Vedas, which were hymns meant to be sung with the utmost precision; anyone singing a false note, warned the Vedas, would "lose his head." The composition of devotional hymns continued first in Sanskrit and then in the modern Indian languages as they evolved.

In the Bhakti movement this use of music reached its highest point. The Bhakti teachers themselves were important composers of hymns, and by composing in the local languages, they made the music accessible to all. The true beauty of Bhakti is found in these hymns. Their rich imagery and symbolism are designed to draw the devotees away from their own world and into that of the divine. These hymns are still sung in homes and temples throughout India and continue to inspire devotees.

Another significant development was the spread of group singing with instruments such as drums and cymbals. In this music, people were encouraged to give themselves over emotionally to the singing and dancing and let their tears flow unrestrained. This helps to develop a form of intoxication through which ecstasy can be experienced. In singing, the beginner initially starts with great enthusiasm. But as they go further, they are overcome by their feelings and are hardly able to utter the words. The songs fill their hearts with love until they become completely silent. Finally, when the last vestige falls, they lose consciousness and are immersed in ecstasy.

The important thing to know is that this ecstasy of Bhakti is not difficult to achieve. Although the ultimate goal of samadhi may require a special effort, the bliss of devotion can be easily achieved by one and all in different degrees. The aspirant may achieve this quite quickly through his or her attempts, but the progress, of course, depends on his or her efforts.

The Union

*Flowers tangled His hair like moonbeams caught
  in cloudbreaks
His sandal browmark was the moon's circle rising
  in darkness.
She saw her passion reach the soul of Hari's mood—
  The weight of joy strained His face; Love's ghost
  haunted Him.*

—Gita Govinda, Twenty-second Song

The final communication of the Bhakta with the Lord is through prayers and meditation. Most sects have short forms of prayers, which the devotee repeats for a certain number of times at fixed hours. There are other, longer prayers in which the common idea is praise of God. Besides these formulaic prayers, devotees can, of course, speak to the Lord in their own words. Prayers fulfill a part of our emotional environment. This has been realized since the earliest religions.

In the human mind, there appears to be a need for something that is greater than ourselves and in which we can seek refuge. Praying fulfills that emotional need and makes our lives smooth. This is similar to the appeal of music or poetry in the human mind, which cannot be denied, but does not seem to offer any rationalization. Hence prayers can be justified even for those who do not accept a personal god. But it is different for Bhaktas, for to them prayers are not an end in themselves but a means to a higher goal.

One prescript of Bhakti is that prayers should never denigrate into begging. We must ask from the Lord nothing else but love for him. There is the story of a man given a single boon who asked for one meal that he could have with his grandchildren on a gold *thaali*. The meaning is that with one boon he was asking for a long life, a happy family, and wealth. In the same way, we should ask for the Lord himself, everything else will come after that. Even asking for salvation and the like is degeneration in Bhakti. Love is always for love's sake. The true Bhakta asks only love from the Lord. The Bhaktas seek no reward for their love; they love because they cannot help loving.

Initially the Bhakta prays in the ritualistic way. Then as the Bhakta is immersed more in God, God seems to acquire a living persona. The Bhaktas feel the presence of God intensely, as someone very near. They then communicate directly to him, and, in their prayers, assume the attitude of speaking to an intimate friend, lover, father, or teacher, asking only for God's love. As their love grows stronger, even these prayers cease and the Bhakta is content to contemplate God in deep meditation. Finally, when Bhakti is ripe, this meditation becomes smooth, like oil flowing from one vessel to another. This is the stage of samadhi, and the Bhakta then loses all consciousness and experiences the bliss of God. Thus the ritualistic prayers deepen into intense spiritual outpouring, which deepens into meditation, and ultimately samadhi.

As they come very near to God, a special relationship develops between the Bhaktas and Ishwar. Bhakti theologians have long recognized that the ways in which Bhaktas love God are often different. In their own methodical way, they have divided this love into different types. These are the attitudes of the *shanta*, the quiet devotee; the *dasya*, the servant; the *sakhya*, the friend; the *vatsalya*, the child; and *madhura*, the lover. The Bhaktas approach God in whichever attitude is best suited to their temperaments. There is no rule as such, and the same Bhakta may cultivate different attitudes at different times. In fact, Bhaktas are often advised to love God in all the different ways, in order to know true love. In the Bhakti movement, the principal stream was that directed toward Krishna, and it is to him that these attitudes find their fullest expression.

The shantas are the quiet devotees. Their love is serene and undisturbed by strong emotions. It is the quiet peaceful love of the complacent person. Such love is said to be inferior in that it would take much longer for such a Bhakta to achieve ecstasy.

The love of the dasyas is different. They feel themselves to be intensely loyal servants of their God. We often find such burning love and faithfulness in the attitude of the servant and master. The servants think only of how to please their master and are on their toes to fulfill his every command. It is as if they have no wishes or desires of their own. It is a love that can be shaken by none, a love that no one else can enter into. Just as the servants of a great person share in their master's glory, so also the devotees remember always that they are the servants of God himself and rejoice in it. The devotees cultivate this love within themselves and take God as their master. In this attitude they can surrender themselves completely to their master, content to leave everything to him with the firm belief that he will take care of them. Their duty is only to serve the master they have pledged themselves to.

Another love is that of the sakhya, or friend. Here God is viewed as a playmate by the Bhaktas. We are all playing in this universe, and our companion now is God himself. The whole world then becomes a playground in which the devotees sport themselves. And in this divine play it is God himself who is the friend of the devotees. There is then no need for them to fear life or to look at it as a stern test. God is not a magistrate frowning on them but a merry playmate who takes them by the hand and leads them in this game. They may then associate him with all the activities of their lives, as one associates a close friend. True friends are the closest to our hearts, and it is they who know more of our inmost thoughts and feelings than anyone else. We give our love unconditionally to our friends, and seek nothing else in return except friendship. This love becomes much more powerful when the devotees take God himself for their friend. No friend can be dearer than God, for God alone is the one who has no interest of his own. He is ready to sport with his devotees and together enjoy this game of life. He will forever support them, and they can then laugh and talk with him, and return his love with their hearts.

Another way to love God is to love him as a child. Parents never waver in their love for the child; it is the simplest and most primitive love in all of us. They will sacrifice themselves a thousand times and brave countless dangers for their child. It is with this primal and possessive love that devotees claim their God. For them, everything else comes second to their God. He has the first right on their lives, and they willingly give up everything to satisfy his demands. Just as parents enjoy the hours spent with their child and can think only of him or her when they are away, so also the devotees' minds are filled with God. They feel restless when they are not in his company. They think of him as someone who needs them, who demands that they give him their love, and they comply. The child is the receiver, and he draws in the love of the devotees until they forget all else.

One more representation of the love for God is madhura, that between the lover and the beloved. This is the highest of all forms of love in Bhakti. In this play of love, God is the eternal male, and all devotees are female. He is the bridegroom to whom the devotees have given their heart's love, and now seek nothing more than to stay immersed in that love. The ideal of this form of love is Krishna, and the greatest Bhakti saints adopted this attitude toward him in their devotion. This is the secret of Bhakti Yoga, for this love is sweeter than any other and the most powerful. As Swami Vivekananda writes, "What love shakes the whole nature of man, what love runs through every atom of his being—makes him mad, makes him forget his own nature, transforms him, makes him either a God or a demon—as the love between man and woman?" The most intense form of love in humans is that of a lover for the beloved, and hence the imagery of the Gopis and Sri Krishna is drawn for the Bhakta.

The story of Krishna is such that each Bhakta may find in him an aspect that enchants the most. There is the story of the love between his mother, Yashoda, and the baby Krishna, and the love between Krishna's boyhood companions, especially Sudama, and Krishna. The love between the master and the student is drawn in the story of Arjuna. But the most celebrated of such depictions is the love between Krishna and the Gopis of Vrindavan.

In the Hindu tradition, Krishna was brought up as a Yadu, a tribe of cowherds on the banks of the Yamuna River, and he lived their pastoral life. The women of the community are eternalized as Gopis, and the Bhaktas sing of the love of the women for Krishna as he beguiles them with his beauty and the enchantment of his flute. They are all mad with love for him, but his true love is Radha, the chief Gopi. The Bhakti hymns depict this love of Krishna and Radha as the ideal for all Bhaktas. The songs of the Gopis convey the keenness, the yearning, and finally the bliss of culmination to form a compelling symbol. Passionate love is said to be even stronger if it is illicit, and hence Radha is depicted as a married woman. The love between Krishna and Radha is the strongest form of love portrayed in Hinduism.

The erotic forms an important part of the symbolism of this love. The desire for sexual union and the bliss of union itself is a pivotal part of love between man and woman. The image would be incomplete if this was not included. There is no prudery in Bhakti, and the sexual act in all its many-sidedness is rendered with great tenderness and sensitivity. But it is important to realize that the whole image was used as a metaphor in Bhakti texts to express this love in its most ardent form. The love of the beloved is a metaphor for love of God, and the desire for the sexual act and the union itself is a metaphor for desire for mystical union with the divine and the fulfillment of this desire.

Like all rituals, this metaphor also has both an outer and inner form. On the outer form, the intense language of the Bhakti saints may appear to depict only the love between two passionate lovers. But as the devotees meditate on this love and draw nearer to God, they realize the inner meaning of the metaphor: that the beloved is the Lord himself. Then they realize the true meaning of this image, and are able to love God with this, the most intoxicating form of love known to us.

The supreme illustration of this love is in the *Gita Govinda*, written by Jayadeva in the twelfth century CE. This book of songs in modern Sanskrit became widespread and rejuvenated the popularity of the lovers' imagery. Partly due to its success, Madhura Bhakti came to be seen as the chief mode of Krishna Bhakti. In this form of love, the devotees assume the attitude of the Gopis of Vrindavan and the same love for Krishna grows in their hearts as is idealized in the Gopis. The love of Krishna and Radha is immortalized in all the Bhakti teachings and in the folklore, arts, and paintings of India. The devotees sing, celebrate, and live this love in all its passion and excitement. The Bhaktas use images from this love and meditate on them, putting themselves in the place of Radha, who is in love with the immortal.

The Bhakta prays to the Lord with the yearning of Radha and seeks the culmination of love in mystical union. It is an all-consuming love, and the Bhaktas know that God will respond to their love as he did for Radha. The Bhaktas become maddened by the love, and forget everything else. They forget their own sexuality and all other narrow conventionalities of society and are immersed day and night in the yearning for the beloved. As the love becomes more intense, the Bhaktas see God more and more clearly, and feel in their heart the thrill of God's love for the mortal. Finally, even God is unable to withstand the power of the Bhaktas' love and grants them their inmost longing. Then the beloved himself comes to the Bhakta, and lover and beloved become one in the most sacred and desired of unions.

The worship of Krishna in his different forms is the most common form of Bhakti mysticism. Krishna is the main *Ishta* of the Bhakti movement, and his worship has given rise to a whole culture of hymns, poetry, and classical arts all over the country, which continues to reverberate as strongly today as in the days when he walked in the groves of Vrindavan.

Besides Krishna, the other important incarnation of Vishnu is Ram. Ram is the hero of the earliest epic, the Ramayana. He is the most perfect of all the conceptions of personal gods in Hinduism. Ram is the supreme embodiment of all the virtues desirable in a human being. He symbolizes courage, chivalry, self-sacrifice, and wisdom. The legends of the Ramayana are replete with stories that describe the behavior of Ram in different situations, and thus provide a guide to the average person in his or her own conduct.

The relation of the devotee with Ram is always one of servant and master. Ram is an ideal of perfection, one that we must all aspire to. Through worship of him, the devotees aspire to achieve this perfection in their own lives, and thus to slowly annihilate their own personalities and finally become Ram themselves.

The path of Ram Bhakti is prevalent mainly in northern India, where it received its impetus with the translation of the Sanskrit Ramayana into Hindustani in the *Ram Charit Manas* of Tulsidas. The work became extremely popular and led to the blossoming of cultural activities such as painting, dance, and music centered on the figure of Ram. Some of the most beautiful hymns in any language are found in his worship. Most festivals and folklore in northern India celebrate Ram and his saga, and thus the ideal is kept always before the mind of each person. In this way, Bhakti is deepened and the devotees approach nearer to their ideal.

But Ram as the ideal of perfection is often found wanting in some aspects. Some Bhaktas are not content with having a God who is perfect and whose perfection itself becomes a difficult barrier. This led to the cult of worship of Hanuman, the monkey God. His tale is told in the Ramayana, where he sided with Ram and was his trusted lieutenant in his struggle. Hanuman embodies Ram Bhakti, he is the *param Bhakta* (ardent devotee) whose only identity is his faith in Ram. At the same time, he is more approachable, with his delightful pranks and escapades. The Bhaktas offer their worship to Hanuman keeping always his ideal of Ram Bhakti before them. In this way, they approach his Bhakti and thus the object of his Bhakti, Ram himself. Thus their way becomes easier.

The other great path in Bhakti, besides Vaishnavism, is Shaivism, the worship of Shiva. Shiva is the third god of the Puranic trinity of Brahma, the creator; Vishnu, the preserver; and Shiva, the destroyer. Vishnu and Shiva have always had their legions of followers, and the conflict between the two groups is legendary in India. The swipes ranged from simple tales by each group showing their own God as superior while the other was shown in a comic and subservient role, to fierce battles where blood was shed.

Shiva is a strange god. He is unlike all other concepts of god in Hinduism. This is explained by historians who assert that he was originally a tribal god who was adapted and absorbed into Hinduism along with the tribes. There are many facets to his imagery, ranging from the lovable common man's God to the austere formless definition of the Advaitists.

The form in which Shiva is most widely known and worshipped is that of a bumbling, ash-smeared, bhang-intoxicated forest ascetic. He is a complete contrast to the pristine holy atmosphere that we usually associate with the imagery of God. Instead Shiva appears as a god of the poor man, a god who is never removed from his followers with the barrier of a faultless bearing. He has within him all the culpability of the common man. He often appears as a comic who is jeered at by arrogant society. Shiva is always referred to in the affectionate "tu" instead of the friendly "tum" or the respectful "aap" when speaking in the second person.

But Shiva is also the destroyer in the cosmic trinity. The forces of destruction can create chaos if they are not controlled, and it is only Shiva who can wield these forces. Because of this, Shiva is considered the most powerful of the trinity. But even he loses control over this power when he is enraged, and then he dances in the mad abandon of the *Tandav Nritya*, which would bring about the annihilation of all of creation. But in the end, it is he himself who prevents destruction from reigning and thus protects the world from slipping into chaos. This terrible power is one aspect of Shiva, and devotees feel safe in the protection of one who holds such power.

The symbol for Shiva used in worship is the Shiva *lingam*. This symbol has had its fair share of controversy, with many modern Indians bristling at any suggestions that it is a phallic symbol. It certainly appears to be connected with the ancient symbolism of the phallus as an organ of creativity and regeneration, and this symbolism that seems so out of place in today's India is perhaps a throwback to the oldest roots of Hinduism. An alternate interpretation is that it is a symbol of a flame or of a mythical pillar that holds up the earth.

Along with his phallic symbol, another intriguing aspect of Shiva worship is his association with the use of *bhang*, or marijuana. Bhang, which grows wild all over India, is an integral part of the armory of Indian ascetics. Shiva, the greatest ascetic, is pictured as being intoxicated with bhang while also drinking wine. No worship of Shiva would be complete without bhang. On the day of his special worship, Shiva Ratri, it is mandatory for even the primmest old lady to join in taking bhang in some form of Prasad (holy offering). Shiva temples are centers where all bhang users gather, and ascetics swear by Shiva's name as they puff away at their *hooka*.

This bumbling, stoned, ash-covered Shiva is also revered as the god who can be most easily pleased by his devotees. Those who desire any boons are advised to worship Shiva. He is called *Bhola-nath*, the innocent Lord, because of this quality. A tale is told of a thief who hid himself on a bilva tree, sacred to Shiva, and during the night idly plucked the leaves of the tree and threw them down, not knowing that there was a Shiva lingam underneath. Even worshipping unaware was sufficient to please the Lord, and in the morning he appeared before the startled thief and granted him boons.

The worship of Shiva is thus straightforward and simple, unlike the often-elaborate rituals of Vaishnavism. The devotee offers a few simple gifts such as milk, sacred flowers, and leaves, and perhaps a bit of bhang, and then proceeds to pray to him and ask for boons. The boon asked for by the true Bhakta is, of course, that of love.

Praying to Shiva does not have any rules; the devotees pray from the heart without a shadow of fear or doubt in their minds. There are tales told of followers quarrelling with Shiva, of getting angry with him and cursing him. Shiva himself receives all this with equanimity, because of his complete love for his followers.

It is perhaps this lack of any sacramental rituals that makes Shiva such an enduring icon in India. He is a god that we need not look up to, a god who is as clumsy and as foolish as we sometimes are. We can build a sense of easy companionship with such a god. Yet this simple god of nature guides us and protects us in our journey through life.

Another conception of Shiva is that of *Ardhanarishwara*, the being who is half-man and half-woman. Shiva's consort is Parvati, who symbolizes the active, creative principle while Shiva symbolizes the potential, inactive principle. This is traced directly back to the Tantric traditions, and even further back to the Samkhya philosophy. Ardhanarishwara symbolizes the union of the opposite dualities, the Purusha and Prakriti of the Tantras, and thus symbolizes all of creation itself. Shiva is worshipped in this form mainly through Tantric rituals.

Shiva is the god of the ascetics of India. The tradition of asceticism is an ancient one. It is the ascetics who are believed to hold the real spiritual power in India, not the priestly class connected with temples and society. The paths followed by ascetics are as different and varied as in the rest of the religion. But the one factor that binds almost all ascetic paths is in the worship of Shiva, although he is conceived differently from Tantric forms to the Advaitic form.

Another conception of Shiva is that of Advaitism. The Advaitists were all Shiva Bhaktas. Shiva is the personal god worshipped by the Advaitists when they practice the path of Bhakti. Shankaracharya himself was a great Shiva Bhakta, and he has several beautiful compositions dedicated to Shiva in his name. In the Advaitic conception, Shiva is conceived as the personification of the formless principle, the absolute. Shiva here is seen in his dualistic avatar, but only as a form to concentrate upon and work toward. He is worshipped through his symbol of the linga and through simple rites of worship.

In this conception of Shiva, the Advaitist draws up the most powerful image of the absolute as seen through the mind, in highly evocative language. The hymns dedicated to Shiva in this tradition emphasize the absoluteness of Shiva, and thus of creation itself. The Advaitist sings, "I am Shiva, I am Shiva." Through the conception of Shiva, the Advaitist is able to focus all the powers of concentration and love in his or her mind on the form of the Lord.

By meditating constantly on Shiva, the Advaitists approach nearer and nearer to the Lord until they achieve merger with him. In the ultimate stage, the Advaitist strikes down even this image and achieves final merger with that beyond both personal and impersonal, the absolute. Thus through their conception of Shiva, the Advaitists press onward toward their goal of samadhi in the absolute. It is in this, the absolute principle of Advaita, that the highest conception of Shiva is reached.

The third important stream of Bhakti in Hinduism is the worship of the Divine Mother. This was mainly a Tantric form of worship, and will be dealt with in the section on Tantricism on page 334.

Traditions of devotion similar to Bhakti in that they hold with the goal of mysticism (the inner experience of the divine) are also seen in other religions, such as Christianity and Islam. Christian mystics describe three stages in the progress of the devotee. First is the stage of preparation, when the ego is uplifted through observance of rites and devotion to the personal god. In the second stage there is ecstatic union or contact, and in the third stage a change in the person, whereby they remain under constant influence of God.

The ideal or Ishta for Christians is Jesus Christ. The story of Jesus Christ is told with infinite tenderness and beauty. In it we find all the highest ideals that inspire man: love, compassion, and, above all, bravery. For the story of Jesus Christ is that of a hero— not a hero of war, but one of love, who sacrificed himself for the whole of humanity. The parallels between the life story of Christ and of Krishna are striking, especially in their births. Both were born in similarly adverse circumstances, under a king who had ordered that all newborns should be killed; both were foretold by angels; and both had ultimate miraculous escapes to return triumphant to the same city. In Jesus Christ, we also find the same ideals of love, in the baby Jesus, and in Jesus as the friend, master, and also, sometimes, as lover.

These different ideals of love were used by various mystics in their praise of the Lord, although perhaps not consciously as in Bhakti. We find in the writings of the mystics the same tender way of seeing Christ as someone intimate; these writings also display different attitudes of love toward Christ. This ideal of a lover is expressed in Christianity as that of the bride waiting for the bridegroom. This idea gained most of its strength in the last five hundred years, and was popularized by mystics like St. John of the Cross, who, in poems reminiscent of Bhakti texts, wrote of the "union with the beloved."

The method of worship used in Christianity was described as prayer and contemplation. In practice, it is often very similar to the meditation of Bhakti Yoga. In the Hesychast tradition, the form of prayer used was to repeat a certain formula, which would eventually lead to ecstasy; for example, "Lord Jesus Christ, Son of God, have mercy on me, a sinner." The Hesychast also developed a form of contemplation that was similar to the Yoga of Hinduism, in which the aspirants were taught to pay attention to their breath and fix their eyes on the middle part of the body. This was derided as "navel gazing" by orthodox theologians and viciously suppressed.

The rites of worship in Christianity are also remarkably similar to Hinduism, especially those of the Catholic Church. The same forms of symbolism are used that portray Christ as someone so close that we can touch his flesh and spirit. Other ideals in Hinduism, such as the detachment of Karma Yoga, are also known in Christianity. But the path to mysticism in Christianity is primarily through Bhakti, and other methods like those of Karma, Jnana, or Raja Yoga are not practiced.

Mysticism was never a central goal in Christianity, because the main force of the religion was in its social reach. But in modern times, where religion is no longer seen as a social duty but rather as an individual faith, mystical traditions are being re-explored, and the rich tradition of Bhakti in Christianity is gaining the upper hand.

In Islamic mysticism too, the same ideals of love are expressed and glorified. The great mystical poet, Rumi, sang his love to his beloved, and prayed for their union. The love for God was expressed in the language of earthly love by several great Sufi poets through allegories. The Arabic poets expressed this love through the love for a young boy, as in India it was expressed as the love for woman. Different allegories were also used, such as the desire of the moth for the candle, and also the symbolism of the wine, the drinker, and the cupbearer.

All Sufis, without exception, expressed their total faith in Allah, and mystical experience was always sought through him. Various means were used to achieve the state of ecstatic union, which were very similar to Bhakti. Many use the repetition of the word Allah, or the formula of profession of faith, which was sometimes accompanied by rhythmic movements of the body. Methods of breath control, up to complete holding of the breath, were also practiced. The dervishes used their rotating dancing movements to the accompaniment of compelling music to reach an ecstatic, trance-like state.

Some sects sought a total surrender to God, by which they left themselves totally to God's will, where even thinking of the next day was considered a fall. A Moroccan sect took this to comfortable heights and refused to work altogether, fearing it would sully

God's day. Music also became an integral part of worship, as also such pre-Islamic practices as lighting of lamps or candles and joss sticks.

The goal in all this was the same: interior knowledge, or love of God, which would bring about a union of lover with the beloved. The final goal was annihilation of one's own qualities and personality. The mystics saw themselves becoming fainter and fainter as godhood rose inside them and completed their final extinction as they "took over the qualities of God."

The Sufi tradition has never been accommodated by orthodox interpretations. The orthodox disagree with such aspects of Sufism as saint worship, the visiting of tombs, musical performances, and the adoption of pre-Islamic and un-Islamic customs. The reformers object to the influences of the monistic interpretation of Islam upon moral life and human activities

Despite being attacked and marginalized, however, the Sufi tradition has always exerted a very strong influence in Islamic society, and it is an indispensable part of the richness of Islamic culture that we see today. Sufism continues to spread its message of moderation and tolerance, and its voice has become even more relevant today to Islamic society.

The tradition of Bhakti is important individually to each of us. It is important not only for its goal of the ultimate mystical experience, but because it imbues the world with God, and thus raises our lives to a divine search. The presence of God so near to us steeps our lives with wonder and fills every single day and every event with the potential for infinite bliss.

Once the Bhaktas have achieved the bliss of God, they achieve complete peace, "the peace that passeth understanding," as the Bible puts it (Philippians 4:7). They have renounced all of their actions to God and live immersed in the deep love for God. They achieve a state of mind in which there are no interests, and hence nothing is opposed to it. They finally achieve the bliss that is our true selves.

Who has not experienced the thrill of loving? But ordinary mortal love is fraught with anxiety and tension, for things of the world are mortal and changeable. But once this love for the immortal is achieved, this love from which springs all other love, then we know the supreme bliss of love. This love, stronger than anything that this world can give us, ties the Bhaktas, maddens them, and fills them with the bliss beyond which there is nothing.

Bhakti teaches us that this divine love exists in this world itself. We have only to find it, and the whole world will be ours. When we see the world in this light, then the world does not scare us anymore. Then it is to us "a mansion of light, here I will sing, eat, dance, and be merry."

II

Raja Yoga

He asks, "which desire of yours shall I sing?"
Because this one who, having this knowledge, sings the Sama,
he is certainly able to fulfil desires by singing.

—Chandogya Upanishad I.viii.9

R
aja Yoga is the path of attaining the mystical experience
by connecting with the absolute power within us. In Raja
Yoga, the source of all the power of the universe is within
us, and the goal of the Yogi is to control and harness his mind and
body so that he can connect with this power. Raja Yoga is the path
normally associated with the word Yoga in India. When someone
is described as following the path of Yoga, it usually means that he
or she is following the path of Raja Yoga.

Yoga is the science of exploring the internal world. A scientist
observes facts of the external world and deduces laws from these
facts. Yogis also observe facts of the internal world, what goes on
in the human mind and its relation to the body, and deduce laws
about the way they work. Countless observers in the world of Yoga
have systematically noted these mind-body events since ancient
times.

When numerous observers have agreed that a certain relation is
correct, it becomes an incontrovertible fact. Because these are the
results of observations by numerous sages, they are not individual doctrines but universal findings, and can be experienced by

anyone following the right method. Yoga can be seen in that sense as an experiment: an experiment of the mind for which the Yogi has described a certain procedure and declared that, if it is carried out, a certain result can be seen. This can then be verified by anyone who follows the methods described by the Yogi.

This is the great strength of Hinduism. Its teachings are not based on belief but on test. Its teachings can all be tested and confirmed by the aspirant. Religions are generally based on doctrinal teachings, and followers are asked to believe in something because someone wiser and greater than them laid down these laws. But Hinduism makes the assertion that the aspirant can test whatever it teaches, and in fact its main purpose is to lead the aspirants to test these beliefs and have them verify the teachings for themselves. True religion will be achieved only when this process is started. Someone who sets out to verify these teachings by following any of the four systems of Yoga is a Yogi.

The systematic technical scriptures of Raja Yoga contain the description of *asanas*, breath control exercises and meditation. Yoga is not simply a meditation technique, though, but an entire school of philosophy. Along with *Samkhya*, it is perhaps the oldest orthodox philosophy in India among the six schools, believed by many to be even older than the Vedantic school. In general, Yoga follows all the doctrines of Samkhya with only one or two minor differences. Its importance is in the method of practice that it developed. The main treatise of Yoga is the "Yoga sutras" of Patanjali. Its date and authorship are disputed, but it is this scripture that defined much of Hinduism and Buddhism.

The Samkhya divides the world into two strict categories: *Purusha*, the male principle, and *Prakriti*, the female principle. Purusha is the conscious principle, and it sets off the unconscious principle into the activity of creation, much in the way a snow-ball sets off an avalanche in a mountain, and becomes connected to it. There is no God in Samkhya, but Yoga accepts a god, although his role and functions are never defined. The Purusha is analogous to the soul, and each living person has his or her own individual conscious entity.

The goal is to achieve the discontinuity of the Purusha from Prakriti, so that consciousness stands alone and is no longer drawn into this chaos. Prakriti here is not just the matter and energy of the universe; it also comprises mental substance. In Samkhya and Yoga, it is believed that the mind unconsciously produces thoughts, sensations, and memories, which are just the workings of the mind. These thoughts, sensations, and memories only become part of consciousness in the conjunction between the Purusha and the mind. Thoughts, sensations, and memories are, as it were, streams of information that are fed into the consciousness.

The mind is considered to have four parts: the *ahamkara* (ego), the *buddhi* (discriminative faculty), the *manas* (mind), and *indriyas* (sense organs). The indriyas, or the sense organs, bring their impulses from the outside to the mind, or manas. At the same time, the manas is also the receptacle for our different thoughts and impressions. All these are then presented to the discriminative faculty, the buddhi.

The buddhi is the intellect, or the decision maker. This is the highest of the mind organs, and it determines what thought or sense organ we are conscious of. Connected to the buddhi is also the ahamkara, or the ego, which gives us our sense of "I"ness. All these are not within the realm of consciousness, but are merely "information processors" as part of Prakriti. The Purusha connects to this information stream, and then we have our human consciousness.

Again, all these are not considered absolute organs, merely a division in terms of psychological understanding of the mind. They are all formed from *citta*, which is the mind stuff, or the material the mind is made of. Citta is hence a part of Prakriti and by itself unconscious. The various "mind organs" are arranged like ripples on the citta. These ripples (*vrittis*) then cast their shadow on the Purusha, which becomes "colored" by them, just as a lake bed is colored by ripples on the water. The mental manifestations, the mind, and so on are the finer or higher manifestations, and the material manifestations, like the body and other objects, are the grosser manifestations of Prakriti. Yoga controls these ripples in the citta and makes the Purusha free of the mind, so it remains as consciousness alone. Because the ripples are formed by factors such as thoughts, sensations, and so forth, by controlling our thoughts and sensations, we can control these ripples and still them, making the Purusha free.

The Yoga philosophy relies on other parts of the Vedas than the Upanishads; it is not a Vedantic (Upanishadic) school (although it is still, of course, a *Vedic* school). Its original philosophy had many inherent contradictions and soon died out, but the Vedantic schools, including Advaita, took up the practice. The duality between a real and existing Prakriti and a consciousness is considered to be a halfway theory and is not accepted by Advaita. The Advaitist pushes beyond this post and achieves the merger with the one unchanged Brahman.

In Advaita, it is the absolute Brahman that is, in the constricted state, manifesting as our individual consciousness, and this constriction is brought about by the senses, thoughts, memories, and so on. (In other words, by the working of the mind.) Thus, we exist on two levels of consciousness: the individual consciousness and absolute consciousness. In Advaita, there is no sharp division between the matter of the mind (the brain) and consciousness. Information is always associated with matter; they are two sides of the same coin. They are two dimensions of differentiation of the same absolute Brahman.

When matter is arranged in such a way that an information flux is produced, individual consciousness is produced. When this information flux becomes still, then the individuality is lost and the individual consciousness experiences the limitlessness of absolute consciousness. Because both the matter and the information flux—the ripples in the chitta—have only an amorphous reality and do not have an absolute existence, the real existence is still the absolute. Neither the matter nor the information flux really exists in the true sense, and all this existence is always the absolute; and hence the absolute reveals itself when the information flux is stilled.

The stilling of the ripples is a necessary part, and this stilling is achieved through the techniques of Raja Yoga, so these methods can also lead to the Advaitic realization. Thus Advaita adapts the practices of Raja Yoga, even while rejecting its theory, and harmonizes them to explain Rajasic samadhi based on its own metaphysical philosophy.

Raja Yoga techniques have evolved over thousands of years, and by following these techniques, the Yogi can obtain total control over both his mind and body. Such control is achieved by sheer force of will power. Normally, we do not have much control over either our body or mind; we are more or less slaves to them. We fall ill, and thoughts and desires come to us unbidden, even when we try to stop them. But Raja Yoga says we can use our will alone to have total control over every aspect of our physical existence.

We can control and feel every part of our body—such as, for example, the beating of our heart. We can also control our minds completely and become aware of all the intricate psychical events going on within that. These are normally at a preconscious level, and through control we can stop all thoughts at will. Once we acquire such control, we have virtually limitless potential.

Yoga believes that all the forces and all the power in the universe are connected directly to us, as all of nature, both matter and mind, is one and only differs in grades (because all are a part of Prakriti). Among these, the mental aspect is highest. Once we gain control over our physical body and then our mental, we have control over all of Prakriti and can achieve anything we want. We acquire the eight powers of the Yogi, to become as light as air, to become invisible, heavy as the earth, and so on, and to make all our desires come true at once. We become virtual gods. But if we remain in the grip of these powers, we still remain on the material plane. The true goal is beyond this: to sever the connection between Prakriti and Purusha, so that the Purusha, the pure consciousness, attains total freedom.

In Advaita, as we come nearer to Brahman, we also come closer to the root of all the energy and power of the universe. All mental and physical existence differentiates from the same root, and once we come to this root, we can have control over everything. The closer we are to samadhi, the greater the power we acquire. But to achieve the final goal, we must give up the temptations of such distractions and press onward towards the end.

The Practice

Now, that light, which shines beyond the whole creation, beyond everything, in the highest worlds which are unsurpassingly good, it is certainly this which is the light within a person.

—Chandogya Upanishad III.xiii.7

Raja Yoga follows the system of practice laid out by Patanjali. It consists of eight steps:

1. Ayam: the ethical don'ts
2. Niyam: the dos
3. Asana: posture
4. Pranayama: breath-control exercises.
5. Pratyahara: mind-cleansing exercise
6. Dharana: concentration
7. Dhyana: unbroken meditation
8. Samadhi: the final culmination.

Ayam and niyam are the system of ethics laid out in the Yoga sutras. They more or less consist of the same ethical rules seen throughout the world. Ayam, the don'ts, are to not tell lies, not kill, not steal, practice continence, and not accumulate more than is necessary. Niyam, the do's, are internal and external purification, contentment, mortification, study, and worship of God.

These ethical rules have a purely practical function: they help in Yoga. There is no moral basis to these rules, as is seen in the Upanishads. Breaking these rules causes "a tying of a knot in the heart," in other words, they lead to physical and psychological problems. This can be understood in terms of modern techniques like the use of lie detectors to test truthfulness. When the subject tells a lie, he has changes in various body functions, like enlarged pupils, a rise in blood pressure, sweating, and so on. Even such small transgressions lead to important changes in the mind and body.

So these ethical boundaries are apparently hardwired into the human body, perhaps during the evolution of living within a social herd, and are common for everyone. Such disturbances in our physiology will naturally be detrimental to the practice of Yoga, and these acts should be avoided. Raja Yoga advises us to act ethically, not on the basis of some arbitrary moral doctrine, but in order to maintain our equilibrium and tranquility.

Yoga believes that following such rules gives us an immense power—not just a moral power, but a psychical power as well. It lays the strictest importance on telling the truth. If we make a promise to do something, we have to carry out that promise no matter what, so that our words do not become false. Yoga says that if we continue telling the truth in this way, a time will come when our will becomes so strong that whatever we say becomes the truth and comes to fruition. Hindu myths are full of stories of sages who have this power of cursing or blessing people and whose utterances or curses are never thwarted.

The most important point among all these is the renunciation of all ties and bonds, including sex. Continence is *the* prerequisite for Yogis, and there is no compromise on this. Without it, the Yogi can never attain success. Yoga believes that there is a certain amount of spiritual energy, *ojas*, in every human, and this energy is to be used during Yogic practice. Sexual activities fritter away this energy and are to be avoided. Even without such theories, it is easy to see that a sexually active life can be very distracting. One cannot attain the single-mindedness necessary for success. Complete continence is demanded, not just in deeds, but also in thought.

This is doubtless one of the toughest demands that can be made on most people living a worldly life. Calls for such forbearance are often ridiculed. People who can renounce the demands of their bodies are said to lack a zest for life or not to be leading a full life. The consternation of most people at such exhortations can be seen in the same light as the slight ridicule with which someone who enjoys his drinks looks upon the teetotaler, or a meat eater looks upon the vegetarian.

It really depends on where we draw the line. We all have to draw it somewhere in order to balance our indulgences with our studies, work, or other social needs. We draw the line at the point that seems the most appropriate to us—for example, in how much we would consider reasonable to drink. Anyone crossing our personal limit seems reckless, and anyone who draws it much tighter than us seems too prudish.

But we tend to forget that others judge us in the same manner. In such cases, those who indulge invariably feel that the sacrificing person is giving up something very important, while the persons who renounce feel that they have acquired a much deeper enjoyment by sacrificing something cruder. A student going out for a party may scoff at someone settling down to study for his exams, yet both give equally valid reasons to themselves for doing their own thing. In the same way, *brahmacharis,* or celibates, also feel they have acquired something much greater by giving up a smaller thing, and, in fact, they actually find their lives as rich and fulfilling as any profligate, and usually far more so.

Along with sexual activity, Yoga also demands sacrifice of all ties and bonds toward society, including family and social ties. They must strictly avoid ownership of any property or wealth. True Yogis must lead lonely lives, and in their search for truth they cannot succumb to simple pleasures like loving and being loved. Not all of us feel a desire for truth so compelling that our worldly ties begin to look like burdens, and unless we have that trait in our character, we can never really break such golden chains easily.

For worldly people, the path that is recommended is the path of Bhakti, and not the high, lonely path of Yoga. Of course, such an extreme course is only the ideal, and meant for very few. We can still do Yoga without going to such lengths, but these exhortations must be kept in mind, and we must try to stay as close to them as individually possible.

Certain practices are also helpful before beginning Yogic exercises. One of the most important things is the practice location. Practice must always be done in the same place, which should be quiet and comfortable. The room should be arranged attractively by keeping it clean and arranging flowers within. Pictures and representations of gods that are dear to us should also be kept in the room, and before practicing every day, we can hold a small *puja* offering flowers and incense. Christians can offer prayers from the Bible, and Muslims can read passages from the Qu'ran. The motive is to bring us into a spiritual mood. By repeating such practices daily, our reaction will ultimately change so that simply entering the room prepares us, and our mood becomes receptive.

The timing of practice is also important. In Yoga, the motive is to achieve stillness. Stillness occurs during moments of change— for example, between inhaling and exhaling during breathing. Similarly, during the day, it is believed there are two moments when everything is stilled: at dawn, when there is change from night into day; and at dusk, from day into night. Such stillness is also present during midday and midnight. These are the four recommended times of Yoga practice. These times are said to last forty-five minutes, and this is considered the ideal length for a session in the beginning. Of course it might not be possible for most of us to practice so often, but we should try to use the dawn and dusk times, which are the most powerful.

Asana

Asana is posture. Asana receives only a brief mention in Patan-jali's Yoga sutras, but it was subsequently built up into an entire system of its own: Hatha Yoga. The posture recommended for yogic meditation is the *padmasana*, a form of squatting with the legs tucked firmly under each other. The aim of this posture is to keep the body as still as possible. Yoga should preferably be done sitting on the floor, and a soft mat can be used for seating. It is useful to keep a small cushion or a folded-up towel for the seat. The spine should be straight and erect, and this should lift up the chest. The flow of energy within the body is along the spine, and this should be unhindered. If our mood is depressed, we find ourselves hunching. Straightening up will immediately help.

During meditation, we should keep a soft smile on our face. In Yoga it is believed that the physical body corresponds to our mental one, and just as an inner happiness makes us smile, smiling will make our mind light. Forcing a smile is one effective way of countering unhappy moments.

Hatha Yoga comprises an elaborate system of asanas, or positions, which are meant to be of physical help. There are hundreds of different postures, and they all have different functions that help different organs and parts of the body. The benefits of this system are only now being rediscovered by scientific methods. These asanas are not directly connected to Raja Yoga.

Pranayama

*It is verily you who move about in the womb as the Lord of
all Creation, and it is you who take birth after the image of
the parents. O Prana, it is for you, who reside with the organs,
that all these creatures carry presents.*

—Prasna Upanishad II.vi

Pranayama is the path to controlling *Prana*, cosmic energy.
Pranayama is described in only one or two sutras, but it developed into a branch of its own. Pranayama soon became such a
powerful tool that the mystical experience could be found through
it alone, though it began as a preparatory tool for Yoga.

Prana is the sea of cosmic energy flowing through the universe.
It is not the actual manifested energy, but the subtle form from
which it is manifested. In Yogic philosophy, all of nature is one,
and there are only different gradations, subtle and gross, of the
basic forces. The energy in the human body is a part of this cosmic
energy, but a finer form of it. Thoughts are the finest form of
energy. There are millions of channels, 720 *lakhs* (an Indian unit
of a hundred thousand), in the human body, and there is a continuous flow of energy, or Prana, through them.

Out of these, the fundamental channels are the two channels
on either side of the spine, the *Ida* and the *Pingala*. The Ida is the
soothing or calming channel and is called the *Chandra* (moon)
channel. It is on the left side and is controlled by breathing through
the left nostril. The Pingala is the exciting or stimulating channel
and is called the *Surya* (sun) channel. It is on the right side and is
controlled by breathing through the right nostril. Normally the
flow of energy within us is discontinuous, and we do not have

much control over it. Through regular practice of Pranayama, we can gradually control it so that the energy flow is harmonious and in equilibrium, and then we have the entire Prana of the universe at our command. There will be no limits to our powers and we will become ever-free.

We are all connected to this ocean of cosmic energy, and we can achieve our desires by drawing from it. The source is infinite, making the potential power in us in infinite. We can be strong or weak, depending on how much of this force we manifest. Powerful persons who influence others draw more upon this energy. We can and do sometimes draw upon this energy, unconsciously, and at these moments we feel a sense of supreme power, as if we can achieve virtually anything. At other times we may feel defeated and weak, and at this moment we are simply not drawing upon this supply. Through Pranayama, we can learn to draw upon this energy whenever we want.

By controlling our breathing, we control Prana. Breathing through the left nostril stimulates the Ida, or the moon channel, and has a calming effect, whereas the right nostril has the opposite effect. Normally our breathing is never smooth or steady, and our Prana is disturbed. The breathing between our nostrils is also unequal at any given time, and this keeps us from attaining equilibrium. By controlling our breathing, we can get control over the Prana in us, and, from there, achieve control over the Prana of the entire universe.

Of course, these theories behind Pranayama are not fully supported by modern science. Some of the observations of our breath have been corroborated by modern physiology. The nose contains erectile tissues, and these have a cyclical flow: one side is swollen when the other is flattened, so we always breathe unequally through the two nostrils. The anatomical cross-section through the spinal cord also corresponds to a great extent to the figure-of-eight diagram of Pranayama, but there is no evidence of a stimulating and a calming side with both sides being functionally the same. There is also no evidence of the Prana channels, although they match well with the Chinese principles in acupuncture, and Prana is also very similar to the Chinese idea of *chi*. It is probable that the idea of Prana, which preceded chi, spread into China through Buddhism.

But even without believing in theories of Prana, the principles behind Pranayama cannot be dismissed. The functions of our body are partly voluntary and partly involuntary—processes over which we have no control, like heart beat, digestion, and so on. Breathing is the most fundamental activity of our body that is controlled both consciously and unconsciously, and by controlling our breath, we can control and harmonize the entire system of our body.

The nose is also directly connected to the brain by its nerves and blood supply. Stimulation of the nose by breathing quite possibly has a direct effect on the brain. It has been proved that the functions of the brain are split into two, and the right brain is the synthetic, subconscious part, which deals mainly with harmonizing our thoughts, while the left brain is the active half, which is more analytical and mathematical. As the functions of the brain are crossed, the right brain controls the left half of the nose and vice versa. It is quite likely that the left nostril will have a calming effect, since it is connected to the right brain, and vice versa. In any case, bringing into equilibrium our breathing should stimulate our brains equally, and thus harmonize everything within us.

A large number of breathing exercises have been developed in Pranayama. Different schools have different forms. Breath consists of three parts: *rechaka* (exhaling), *puraka* (inhaling), and *kumbhaka* (the stationary phase in between). In Pranayama, kumbhaka is the most important phase. The aim is to prolong kumbhaka when all the processes of the body are in equilibrium and stilled.

The two main ways of doing this are described in the Patanjali Yoga sutras. The first is forcefully holding the breath for a certain period, which is determined by the ratios of the three phases. This is stressful and requires a great deal of effort. Only someone who is totally devoted to Yoga can do this. The second is the process of meditation, when meditation on something pleasant is done during kumbhaka so that it becomes prolonged automatically without stress. This is the recommended path for all.

The main exercise of Pranayama is *nadi suddhi*. In Raja Yoga, it is recommended that nadi suddhi be done for six weeks to six months to purify the system, before going for meditation. But Pranayama has developed in such a way that nadi suddhi alone can bring on the mystical experience, in conjunction with meditation. There are also a wide variety of pre- and post-nadi suddhi exercises to be performed.

In nadi suddhi the aspirant, after going through the preliminary calming exercises, sits in the padmasana posture. By holding the right hand in a special way, the right nostril is closed, and breath is slowly and continuously exhaled through the left nostril. Once the entire breath is expelled, meditation is done by visualizing an effulgent lotus between the eyebrows or the heart and imagining that, at this time of kumbhaka, it is giving out and filling the body with an intense bliss. Alternately, meditation is done by visualizing the symbol of "Om" in the mind. In fact, meditation can be done on anything that is ennobling and brings bliss. Christians, for example, can meditate on the form of Christ.

The breath is to be held for only as long as it remains comfortable. Air is slowly breathed in through the left nostril; then the left nostril is closed, while breathing air out through the right. When the breath is fully expelled, meditation is done again during kumbhaka. Then air is breathed in through the right. This completes one cycle of nadi suddhi. Three, six, or nine cycles should be done during one session, with four daily sessions. This is done regularly, until the mind feels strong enough to begin the meditation process of Raja Yoga.

In this method, meditation is only done during the kumbhaka of exhalation, when it is more comfortable. The emphasis should be on comfort, and breath should never be held by force. The process of lengthening of kumbhaka will happen automatically over time. During this phase, one should imagine the body being filled and lifted up with an intense bliss. Bliss or ecstasy is an actual physical sensation, and it can be visualized as a golden effulgent light that fills the body and mind. There is an immense sense of bliss rising up and filling the mind and body, like a glow of delight that uplifts and lightens the body, until one is conscious of nothing but intense happiness. It may sometimes be felt as a light filling the body, or rising up as an intense, "touchable" bubble of ecstasy.

It is interesting that this sensation of bliss is often felt quite early on by the aspirant. Once it is actually felt, the aspirant has an idea of what true bliss is, and this makes his or her belief unshakeable. Even the briefest touch of such bliss is enough to change one's faith. Different physical changes are also said to occur in the Yogi. The mind becomes light, happy, and refreshed; the voice becomes pleasant. One comes to have a sort of power, and everyone becomes attracted to such a person. It is said strange events may occur: one hears beautiful sounds like bells at a distance, or sees everything glowing in a strange and beautiful light. These psychic events may be due to subjective belief, but they are of great importance because they encourage the pupil.

There are also preparatory exercises for nadi suddhi. One of these is the *kapalabhatti*, in which, after sitting in the padmasana, the hands are closed into fists and the knuckles pressed against each other at the level of the abdomen. After this, the aspirant exhales very forcefully and shortly with his whole abdomen and chest, while letting the incoming breath come in automatically and quickly, and then breaths out again at once, so that the whole breathing process is like a bellows. This is done with forty breaths at a time. Only at the end is the breathing allowed to stop and kumbhaka is attained. This stimulates the whole mind and body and readies it for the further exercises.

After nadi suddhi, we should try to calm ourselves down. One exercise for this is the *sitkari*. In the padmasana posture, air is sucked in slowly through the mouth by forming the lips into a whistling shape, and then exhaled slowly through the nose. The effort is to concentrate on the cooling feel of the breath in the mouth, and the warm feel on the upper lip during exhalation.

Another useful general Pranayama exercise is the *Sukha* Pranayama. This is a very simple exercise and can be done either in the sitting or standing position, as long as the spine is straight. The breath is exhaled slowly and deeply through both nostrils as far as comfortable. During kumbhaka, the mind should concentrate on a happy thought, which could be anything: a loved person, a picture, a party with friends, even a risqué joke—anything that fills the mind with delight and happiness. Then the breath is again inhaled slowly. This exercise, done regularly, makes the person's mind happy and relieves stress and tension.

Pranayama is a vital part of Raja Yoga and must be done before commencing meditation. There are various techniques for the exercises, and these have to be learned practically under the direct supervision of a teacher. Just as no one should try to start something like aerobic exercises by reading from a book, it is important to have a teacher for the finer details. But once it is started, almost everyone will feel the direct benefits of Yoga in the body.

Pranayama makes the body light, healthy, and attractive. Besides these physical effects, there are also the benefits to the mind, which becomes much stronger, calmer, and happier. Even if it is not followed through to the mystical experience, Yoga exercises should at least be used for these practical benefits.

Pratyahara

In this exercise, the aim is to understand our mind and its workings so that we can gain control through meditation. In Pratyahara, the effort is to study the flow of the stream of consciousness, slow it down, and eventually bring it to a standstill.

Pratyahara consists of sitting in the padmasana posture and simply observing our minds. As we sit quietly, we can see that thoughts are an intense and dizzying flow. The first step is to try to observe this flow without getting caught up in it. We simply let the thoughts come into our minds and flow through without trying to stop or control them.

In the beginning we will find an immense number of thoughts coming in, remaining for a brief second, and then giving way to the next. It is compared to the process of cleaning a pot, where the water is allowed to flow through it for some time so that it gradually becomes clean. When we observe the thoughts, we distance ourselves more and more from them and come to realize that we are separate from them. In this way, we come to an understanding of how our minds work, and free ourselves from the control of our thoughts. As we sit observing our thoughts without getting caught up in the flow, the flow will gradually slow down, and ultimately stop. Pratyahara is mandatory before starting the next phase of Yoga.

Dharana, Dhyana, and Samadhi

The earth is meditating as it were. The intermediate space is meditating as it were. The heaven is meditating as it were. The mountains are meditating as it were. The oceans are meditating as it were. The gods and humans are meditating.

—Chandogya Upanishad VII.vi.1-2

These three steps are continuations of one another, and they are the final steps leading to the culmination in the mystical experience. They are each different steps in meditation. *Dharana* is concentration, *dhyana* is absorption, and *samadhi* is the final single-mindedness. In dharana, we try to focus our minds on a single object or thought. When our minds are absorbed fully in this single thought and there are no other thoughts in it, it is called dhyana or dhyan, and when we go beyond all thoughts, it is called samadhi. Remaining in perfect concentration for twelve seconds is one dhyan, and twelve such dhyans is samadhi. There are various stages of samadhi of higher or lower grades, and it is when all the restraining effects of thoughts are eliminated that we obtain the final Nirvikalpa Samadhi of Advaita.

Dharana, or concentration, simply means thinking intensely

about something. Suppose we fix our mind on some object and call this thought A. Then we find that, as we are in meditation, various other thoughts keep coming in. As soon as we recognize that other thoughts have come in, we again bring our minds back to A. This can be written graphically as:

A-A-B-C-A-B-C-D-A-P-Q-R-A-H-I-A-A-A-J-K-A-A . . .

When our minds have only the one thought, A-A-A-A-A . . ., it is called dhyana. This is like the smooth flow of oil from one pot to another, without any disturbances in between. Ultimately when the mind remains in dhyana for a long time, we will reach a stage beyond all thoughts, and this is called samadhi.

The objects of meditation in Yoga are varied, and the Yogi chooses the object that he or she finds most comfortable. Some of the commonly used objects are parts of the body, such as the navel or the space between the eyebrows; a burning candle; or a holy object, such as a person or some symbol. There is no religious or cultural imperative in the object of meditation; Yoga does not depend on a particular system of belief or scripture. We may belong to any religion and have an Advaitic, qualified monistic, dualistic, or even atheistic conception. Raja Yoga is concerned solely with the body and the mind. It is not a religion as such but more of a scientific effort. We can use its methods, regardless of our prior beliefs.

The object of meditation need not be an object but can be a single thought, like a short prayer or a mantra. In India, it is often a name of God, and one of the important functions of a guru is to give this holy name to the aspirant.

One of the most important symbols used in this way is "Om." Om is considered to be a holy symbol of the Brahman. In Yoga, words are considered to be of elemental importance, and Om (pronounced AAOUM) contains the essence of all words because it uses the entire vocal apparatus. It is considered the origin of the Christian "amen" and the Islamic "amin." Om has acquired a deep significance in Hinduism, and it is the main object used in meditation.

When the mind goes beyond thoughts of an object and captures its essence, it is called a *samyama*. This is done by meditating on a specific object. Through samyama, the Yogi can gain immense powers. By understanding and fusing with the essence of something, we can have power over it. Psychical activities are considered the finest form of existence of Prakriti, and when the mind itself grasps a quality, the physical body follows suit. Literally infinite powers are promised to the Yogi making samyama on different things. Some of the promised powers are the strength of an elephant (by making samyama on an elephant) and knowledge of the world (by focusing on the sun). By conquering his body he can become light as air, float on water, become invisible, and more.

But all such powers are said to be useless in Yoga. The powers achieved in the initial stages are to be refused. This is somewhat like the powers offered to Jesus by the devil. The goal is to go beyond them all and obtain the ultimate mystical experience: complete freedom from this manifold reality. This is the final stage, Nirvikalpa Samadhi of Advaita. As the mind becomes more and more concentrated, the thoughts become finer and finer. After remaining in dhyana for a long time, the thoughts become so faint that finally they cease altogether, and the stage of samadhi is reached. In this the mind has achieved complete stillness, and there is no movement.

This is the final stage, when the ultimate realization is gained. What the mind experiences during this stage can never be described.

With the cessation of all thoughts, the individual consciousness has died out, and consciousness now exists on its natural plane: the plane of absolute consciousness. This is the plane of existence of Brahman. This is the goal of all Yoga.

Although the philosophy of Yoga has died out, the immense possibilities opened up by its system of practice has ensured that its techniques will live on, and it has found its greatest strength from its use by the Vedantic schools in their mystical search. Raja Yoga has now come to mean many different things within India itself. But for the Advaitist, it is one of the ways to Nirvikalpa Samadhi, and knowledge and practice of Raja Yoga is part of the Advaitic path.

Tantricism

Hari Om! Then, in this small lotus like dwelling of the heart that is within the city of Brahman that is our body, there is a small space. That which exists in this space is to be known. That indeed has to be enquired into for realization.

—Chandogya Upanishad VIII.i.1

Tantra is not one of the six orthodox schools of Hinduism but is an *agama* path, as it quotes for its authority not the Vedas but its own subsidiary texts, which are from a later date. Its doctrines and practice have influenced every branch of the religion, and its rituals now occupy a prominent place in Hinduism.

The philosophy of Tantricism draws largely on the metaphysics of the Samkhya and Yoga schools. We have here the same male-female duality, which is called Shiva and Shakti. The play between the two resulted in the formation of the world, and everything in it is the conjunction of the two. But there is an important difference. In Samkhya, the female principle Prakriti is considered an inert and unconscious principle; it is set into the motion of activity by Purusha, the male principle, which is the active, conscious principle, although it is itself motionless.

In Tantra, Shakti has a much more important role to play. Nature is not simply an unconscious principle but an active creative power, the Mother Goddess. The Mother Goddess holds all the power of the universe, both creative and destructive, and she actively creates the world by herself. The Purusha or Shiva is a passive principle, conscious but serene, watching the play of Prakriti. The world arises from the union of Purusha and Prakriti.

The mystical goal here is not the divorce of the subject and the object, consciousness and nature, but the state of harmonious union of Purusha and Prakriti, to perfectly balance the force of active creation and motionless consciousness within us. This perfection of male-female union is often portrayed as Ardhanariswara, the God who is half-male and half-female. All Tantric rituals are directed toward achieving this perfect harmony within ourselves.

Because she holds both creation and destruction in her hand, Shakti is often portrayed as capricious and whimsical. She is portrayed as a cruel destroyer when she deals out death and as a loving mother when she demonstrates fertility. But this is a false understanding of nature. Nature itself is above cruelty and kindness, destruction and creation, death and life. These are but two sides of the same coin and must necessarily coexist. It would be naïve to see nature as benevolence only.

Because of this duality of creation and destruction, the rituals used to worship Shakti are also often strange, calling for blood sacrifices and magic chants to please her, along with offerings of flowers and sandalwood. Shakti is worshipped in various forms, most commonly as Kali, the dark, bare-breasted goddess, who wears a necklace of human skulls around her neck and carries a decapitated head in her hands. Kali is worshipped not as a benign, munificent god but as a god who can be both bountiful and cruel. She is also worshipped as Mother Bhairavi, the patron saint of wars, and is worshipped in this form by soldiers and all who want her power, including *dacoits* (robbers). Durga is another form of Shakti, when she is seen as the repository of the powers of all the gods. Her power is used for the protection of the universe. One of the most important of her forms is as Mother Kamakhya.

Tantricism is one of the oldest systems of Hindu practice. It continues to be prevalent throughout the country, but its main center was in eastern India. According to Tantric mythology, Shakti was embodied as Rati, the consort of Lord Shiva. Due to social conflict, she was killed while visiting her father. Shiva was pushed into a terrible anger, and he destroyed her father. Unable to give her up, he carried her body on his shoulders and raged in fury throughout the world, bringing about tremendous destruction. The world was in danger of being annihilated. The other gods, to calm Shiva down, began hacking away at Rati's body, and parts of her fell to the ground. Only when her body had been completely removed did Shiva become calm. The points where Rati's body fell down are the main centers of Tantricism, and important Tantric temples arose at these points.

The point where Rati's reproductive organ fell down is considered the most powerful of all Tantric centers, as this was the source of her regenerative powers. This is the temple of Kamakhya in northeastern India, which is the center of Tantricism in India. In Tantra mythology, Kamakhya is the source and origin of all creation. The temple has a long history dating back to prehistoric times, and there are many myths connected to it. It is one place where animal sacrifices are still carried out daily, including bull sacrifices. A little higher up is the block where, in ancient times, humans were also sacrificed. There is no idol of a deity; instead, the center of the temple has a small, dark, natural cave where there is an ever-flowing spring, and its source is considered to be the source of the Mother Goddess.

The power of the goddess Kamakhya rules over Assam, and during the days of *Saat*, when the goddess menstruates, no lamp of worship is lit among the Assamese people, and no farmer will plough his land, because the goddess is not ready. Only when the days are over do the celebrations begin as the goddess regains her reproductive powers. Tantricism once dominated the lives of the people, but the excesses of the system led to a wave of reaction, and ultimately the Vaishnava saints, including Sankardeva in Assam, waged a long war against it. Today it survives mainly as an appendage to mainstream Hinduism, which adheres to the Upanishads.

The practice of Tantricism has a lot in common with Raja Yoga. Here too we have the breath channels, Ida and Pingala, on two sides of the spine. In the middle of this is the channel *Susumna*, the main channel, which is normally closed. In Tantricism there are also six plexuses along this channel, at the levels of the base of the spine, the reproductive organ, the navel, the heart, the neck, and the eyebrows. Each of these is visualized like a lotus.

A lotus is peculiar in that when it is in bloom, it closes at sunset every day and reopens at dawn the next day. This analogy is used in Tantra to visualize the re-blossoming of the lotuses in the spine, which each symbolize a particular power. At the base of the spine in each human being lies his psychical powers and his powers of spirituality, and this is drawn in the symbol of the *Kundalini*, the coiled serpent. Normally the Kundalini lies dormant at the base, and the goal of Tantra is to awaken this Kundalini and make it rise up through the channel of Susumna, awakening each lotus in its way, until it metaphorically bursts out through the top of the head, at the moment of mystical experience.

The rituals used for this awakening of the Kundalini are varied, and among the most discussed is undoubtedly the sexual rituals connected to Tantricism. In India, however, the word Tantric conjures up not the image of a sexual deviant, but a fierce, wild-eyed, ash-covered *sadhu* with an array of chants and magical powers. Like the Samkhya, Tantra believes in the power of words over everything else, and if certain words are chanted correctly, they can make all kinds of things happen. Hence a secretive world of mantras evolved in Tantricism, and adherents claim that, with the right ingredients, chanting of the mantras gives a person limitless power.

It is a common practice in some parts of the country to convince a Tantric to perform his rituals and chants to ask for something, and these rituals demand some rather unusual practices. There is even the occasional human sacrifice in the heart of the country. A more well-grounded use of mantras is in meditation, when the aspirant uses the repeated chanting of a particular mantra to obtain a focused mind, and finally to experience mysticism. The pronunciation of the words is given great importance. By meditating on mantras in this way, the Tantric acquires immense powers, but the true goal is the mystical experience.

Sexual rituals form a very small part of Tantra, but they have always, quite understandably, evoked a great deal of interest. Sex is a part of Hinduism in both the Bhakti path and Tantra. In Bhakti, sexual language is used only as a *metaphor* to give strength to the evocation of love for God. The lover here symbolizes God, and the sexual union symbolizes mystical union. In Tantra, however, sexual activity is actually used as a ritual to obtain the mystical experience.

The theory behind this is that sexual activity is believed to stimulate the Kundalini and lead to its awakening. The effort is to maintain a high state of arousal during sex without actual culmination, and in such a state it is believed that the Kundalini is aroused and ascends up the spine. Some elaborate descriptions of sexual rituals are given that apparently help in this mystical path. These rituals were never completely accepted, and it is unlikely that they were ever really used. The sexual aspect of Tantric practices was almost completely forgotten in India until the Tantric texts were translated. It certainly seems very unlikely that such passions will help in spiritual growth, although they might be fun to try.

A more common and orthodox way of arousing the Kundalini in Tantra is through meditation. After sitting in the recommended posture, the aspirants begin meditation on the base of the spine at first, where they visualize the coiled-up Kundalini. As they meditate, a sensation of heat is usually felt in this area. The Kundalini is pictured to be slowly uncoiling and then rising up the spine. As it touches each lotus, the closed-up lotus unfurls and blooms in effulgent light. In this way, the Kundalini rises up until it finally goes out through the top of the head. As meditation is done regularly, the rising of the Kundalini is said to be actually felt as a tactile sensation, and the unfolding of each lotus gives Tantric powers, until the final freedom of the powers gives the mystical experience.

Another important form of Tantric practice is the use of Pranayama in combination with meditation. As Tantricism came to be more generally accepted, it accommodated techniques of Raja Yoga, which was also, in turn, deeply influenced by it. At the present time, both in Raja Yoga and Tantra, a common technique of combining Pranayama with Kundalini meditation is used rather than the earlier, pure forms. The synthesis of the two techniques has led to a powerful form of Yoga that uses the strength of both the systems.

In this form, the Pranayama exercises are done in the same way, but during kumbhaka, instead of meditating on other objects like Om, the aspirant meditates on the Kundalini, and then visualizes the Kundalini rising up through the lotuses as in Tantra. As it rises up, it fills the body with immense bliss. By meditating this way, the kumbhaka can be prolonged easily and naturally. Through this meditation technique, the powers of both these forms of Yoga are combined and expressed in the same exercise.

Tantricism suffers from all the doctrinal weaknesses of qualified monism. Its strength lies in the harmony it has achieved with nature and its idolization of the female creative principle. Its beliefs and practices have touched all aspects of Hindu spiritual life, and as new movements develop all over the world emphasizing a return to Mother Nature and the concept of earth as a goddess, it is likely to become more prominent.

Among all the systems of Yoga, Raja Yoga appears to be the most entrancing. This is because it promises us the ultimate goal based solely on our willpower. If we can dominate our minds and bodies enough, we will have achieved the state of mysticism. Other Yogas depend on various factors, like discrimination or faith, and promise a long and hard struggle. But in Raja Yoga, those with enough strength of will can rapidly gain mental control and achieve samadhi very quickly.

The religion or faith of a person is of no consequence for this path; the only thing necessary is willpower. The exercises also appear very simple, and can be picked up in a matter of weeks, if not days. But upon practice, we might find that few of us have that immense strength that is required to achieve the goal of the system. Still, Raja Yoga teaches us the means to achieve control over our body and minds, and even when the goal is yet to be reached, the strength that it provides us will undoubtedly help us in other facets of life.

Karma Yoga

This space within the heart is as vast as that space outside.
Within it indeed are included both heaven and earth, as also fire
and air, both sun and moon, lightning and stars. Whatever this
one has here and whatever he has not, all is included in That.

—Chandogya Upanishad VIII.i.2-3

Karma Yoga is the path of Yoga that achieves mystical knowledge through the work done in day-to-day life, by doing one's duty and work in such a way that the inmost knowledge comes through. Karma means "work," or "action." It is also used in a particular sense when defining the law of Karma, which states that we always receive the results of our actions: good results for good actions and bad results for bad actions. The description of such a law is also usually tied up with the ancient Hindu belief of reincarnation, in which it is used to mean that our Karma will determine the kind of body we get in the next life. But in the context of Karma Yoga, Karma is simply used to denote action.

Karma Yoga is concerned with the correct way of doing work. It is based on the teaching that if we do our work in a dispassionate manner, we will be able to achieve an inner tranquility in life until, finally, we achieve complete liberation from all of life's temptations and attain the inner mystical wisdom of the absolute. It sets out to teach what our duties are and how we should perform them to attain this sense.

Karma Yoga is the path to be followed by those who cannot or do not abandon a worldly life, yet are filled with the thirst to have mystical knowledge. If we live in the world, we are perforce bound to do work. We have to work simply to earn a living for ourselves and for those for whom we care. Our circumstance in society also leaves us with many duties at a social level. As long as we live in society, we are forced to do this work. Only when we can renounce everything will we be free from work.

Karma Yoga teaches us how to do this work in such a way that, even by working, we are led closer to the truth of Brahman. Normally, when living in society and being engaged in its various activities, we find that life gradually pulls us down to the lower levels, and so we are not able to acquire true mystical knowledge. A thousand joys and sorrows pummel us every moment of the day, and we are torn apart by success and failure, by regrets for the past and forebodings for the future, and so on. It appears almost impossible to hold on to our search for true knowledge while at the same time living amidst such storms. But this ability can be gained through Karma Yoga.

Karma Yoga alone is sufficient to lead us to the path of mystical knowledge. But in practice, it is one of the four paths that are meant to be followed together by the aspirant. Karma Yoga acts as the base for the aspirants of all the other paths of Yoga also. Except for a small few, even those who follow the paths of Raja, Jnana, or Bhakti Yoga have to live in society and are unable to follow the path of strict renunciation. In that case, all their efforts would be in vain if they do not know the secret of work, as worldly duties are bound to lead them away from any inner knowledge.

These paths demand that the aspirants keep a distance from life and are not suitable for the householder. It is also true that very few of us can feel that such a path of renunciation is actually necessary and not a retreat from our responsibilities. Through Karma Yoga, we can follow these paths even while living in society and performing our obligations. We can ensure not only that our personal and social duties do not lead us away, but that they in fact help us to acquire the truth.

This is the great strength of Karma Yoga: it promises realization to all. It elevates and ennobles life, and it shows us that there is no need to abandon the world and live in a forest in order to acquire knowledge. Because of Karma Yoga, the other paths of Yoga do not remain an exclusive preserve of ascetics, but are open to all.

In a larger sense, Karma means not just the activities in the world but also the smallest of actions, such as breathing and eating. All these are activities too, and even a *rishi* in the forest cannot avoid them. Hence Karma Yoga is essential even to the man of renunciation, who is in a way indulging in action as much as someone in society.

The secret of doing work in Karma Yoga is the adage "work for work's sake." This means that no matter what work we are doing, whether it is a daily desk job at the office, painting a picture, or carrying a load, all our efforts and our whole mind should be bent to the job alone. No other thought or action should occupy us at that moment. We must not be thinking of the end result of the work, the benefits that we will get from it, and so on. Our entire concentration, our whole life at that time, consists of that job alone.

When we can do work in this way, Karma Yoga says we obtain complete detachment from work. This is the other corollary of working, according to Karma Yoga. When the work is finished, we can get up from the job without thinking about it for a moment more. When we have finished one task, we will have immediately started another task, even if it is something as simple as relaxation. But even then, our minds would be on that moment alone, engaged only in doing whatever we are doing to relax.

Hence we are detached from work in the sense that we are not mental prisoners of our work; our thoughts relate only to whatever we are doing at that moment. When our work attains such perfection, we obtain liberation from the day-to-day drudge of our daily lives and ultimately attain freedom within life itself. Through this, mystical knowledge is attained, even while leading a full working life in society.

Normally, we work without any real concentration. Most of the time we are thinking about something else—usually the result the work will bring—or our concentration is elsewhere and we are thinking of other things. This prevents us from enjoying the work that we are doing. Our work then becomes drudgery, and we are torn by anger and frustration, which only makes the job worse. This becomes a vicious cycle, and life becomes an inescapable trap.

The results of work can never be predicted. There are far too many factors that impinge on every aspect of life. Even when we put our best effort into work, it might not lead to success because of factors beyond our control. If work was done only in anticipation of its benefits, then it might lead to great frustration. Failure can demoralize us, and then work will seem distasteful and impossible. At the same time, a great success can give us intense happiness, but this happiness is bound to be short-lived, as with everything in life. Working in this way, thinking only of the results, we will find our lives affected by a succession of success and failure, by pleasures and disappointments. We will be caught firmly in the grip of *maya* and find our goal of freedom slipping further and further away.

But when we can do work for work's sake only, when our minds are not troubled by anything other than doing the work as perfectly as we can, according to Karma Yoga, work cannot imprison us. Even when living an intensely busy life, we can still maintain a detached attitude to life and struggle onward for freedom.

Karma Yoga also says that when we work without attachment, we produce the best work. This is the most important aspect of Karma Yoga for our practical lives, because it gives us a guide to being the most efficient producer and supplier of work. Normally, when we are thinking of other things, we naturally cannot give full attention to work, and our work cannot be as efficient.

But if we can avoid thinking of anything else, if we can avoid thinking even of how and why we are doing the work and how it will benefit us, and concentrate instead on doing whatever we are doing to the best extent possible, then the work that we produce is naturally of a far higher order. It is paradoxical that by not thinking of the results, we obtain the greatest results. We always want to produce the best work possible, but because we are unable to be detached from the work, we are led away from the path of Yoga, and we do not attain the success we are capable of.

In this principle, Karma Yoga differs from many modern-day coaches, who teach their wards to visualize the final point of success, of crossing the finishing line first and so on. In Karma Yoga, such visualization of the result is not advocated and instead, according to its principles, the trainee should concentrate on the particular training that he or she is receiving at that moment without thinking of the final result.

Another question that might arise is whether we really want to attain the calmness of a Karma Yogi. It is true that our lives are full of both pleasures and disappointments, but do we really want a life with neither? Success and failure are a part of life, and most of us would much rather face the rough and tumble of such a life than lead one that is flat and emotionally dead.

But this is a wrong way of understanding the ideal of Karma Yoga. Karma Yoga says true happiness comes to us only when our minds are free. We can find true happiness only when we are not bound down by worries of our work. Here work is not just the job we do for our living; it encompasses everything in our lives, the way we raise our children and fulfill our responsibilities to those we love and cherish, and even our simple sensory acts such as eating and drinking. All this work can be truly enjoyed only when done in the spirit of detachment.

The work done normally, with tremulous worrying about the results and a thousand other things, does not give us true happiness, because we are hardly enjoying it at that time. The successes that we obtain are also short-lived and inadequate, because they are tied to a thousand other worries and hopes, and thus it is not true happiness. In Karma Yoga, true happiness comes when we are not tied to this wheel anymore, when we are free from it all with nothing affecting us.

When we reach such a stage, our each work gives us intense happiness; our every work is a worship and triumph. It is not that we are to abandon all passion in life; instead, we are to put intense passion into each moment. Each moment of doing work is a celebration. This is true happiness. The Karma Yogi's life is not that of a zombie but a life of continuous fulfillment, a life that is liberated at the same time. By abandoning the results, such Yogis leave behind all the successes and failures, the mundane joys and disappointments, and in return they receive a sense of bliss far greater than anything that can be achieved through a worldly life.

For a Karma Yogi, all actions are of equal value. All work we are called upon to do in life requires the same intense concentration. There is no higher or lower work in Karma Yoga. The liberation that can be achieved or the happiness that work brings is not dependent on the kind of work that a person has to do, but instead on the way he or she is doing that work. If it is done in the true Karma Yoga spirit, all work can bring us toward the goal of freedom.

The situation that Karma Yogis are in or the work that they are doing does not change their attitude to the work. A Karma Yogi can achieve the same intense concentration while working in a busy life as they can in the middle of a desert. Once the secret of work is learned, it becomes a habit, and it rules over every aspect of a person's life. It also directs every small action throughout the day, and every single moment of the day can be a step further toward liberation.

> *From every rule of thine, O King Varuna, set us free;*
> *From whatever oath by the waters, by the kine,*
>   *by Varuna, we have sworn,*
> *From that, O Varuna, set us free.*
>
> —Sama Veda., 1.3.11

The attitudes people take toward work are widely varied. Hinduism classifies these general attitudes into three different categories: *Rajas*, *Tamas*, and *Sattva*. These define the emotional character of a person. Tamas is the negative reaction, such as laziness and selfishness. Rajas is the aggressive reaction, the "over-positive," as in arrogance and anger And Sattva is the perfectly balanced reaction, like unselfish acts and kindness. Sattva is not the equilibrium of Rajas and Tamas but a different category in itself. In Karma Yoga, Sattva is the attitude that a person should practice toward all situations in life.

Tamasic persons are those characterized by laziness, fear, and obsessive selfishness. It is seen in the deception of others, telling lies, delighting in the fall of others, and sullen cruelty. Rajasic persons are characterized by arrogance, anger, and indifference to the plight of others. This is demonstrated in impatience and restlessness, consuming passions, destructiveness, and instability.

Sattvic persons are those of the greatest character, characterized by pure unselfishness, kindness, and a spirit of self-sacrifice. They are steady, persevering, and truthful, neither angry nor submissive, neither violent nor lazy, neither unkind nor arrogant. Sattvic persons are always cheerful, happy, and sweet and caring towards others. They give unconditional help whenever it is sought and are guided by uncompromising honesty. It is this attitude that is sought after in Karma Yoga. Karma Yogis are not required to be unemotional and cold; rather, they should be characterized by the lightness and warmth of a Sattvic person in all their reactions to life.

Of course, these three traits are usually not found in a pure state in any action or person. All actions combine these three traits, but only one trait dominates. Similarly, in general, no person is purely Rajasic, Tamasic, or Sattvic. Everyone has all three elements combined and present in every situation, and the dominant trait in their character depends on the person. But in those persons of the highest order, the Sattvic character dominates totally.

Sattvic persons are indifferent to the praise or criticism of others, and they are not affected by the nature of the results of their work. They accept both success and failure with equal grace and continue with their undaunted perseverance. In Karma Yoga, it is said that no work can have a purely good or a purely bad result. In every situation in life, something that is a benefit at one point is bound to cause harm at another point. We have no control over this; in fact, we are unable to understand all the ramifications of our actions, many of which will produce results at a much later date, in totally unexpected ways. So we cannot call any result purely good or bad, as all results are a mixture of both these elements. Once this is understood, there will not be any preoccupation with the results of our actions; we will be content as long as we have given the work our greatest effort.

When we are preoccupied by results, we are torn apart by bad outcomes and elated by good outcomes. But we are equally deceived in both and therefore likely to set ourselves up for some paradoxical reactions at a later stage, when the delayed ramifications of our actions bear their fruits. The only solution for avoiding this rollercoaster of emotions lies in the path of Karma Yoga.

In all these injunctions, the question naturally arises as to what our duty is and what sort of work we should be doing. Karma Yoga says our duty is whatever we find in our particular position and situation in life. But often enough in life, we find that our duties in different spheres clash with one other. Sometimes an act that is appropriate in one situation might turn out to be wrong in another, or the duty enjoined by society in a particular sphere might seem unacceptable to us.

These are everyday problems faced by all of society because of its conflicting nature, and it is difficult then to know how to act. Karma Yoga lays down a general rule to guide us in all such situations: perform that action which is Sattvic and avoid that which is Rajasic or Tamasic.

Sattvic actions are purely unselfish, and such actions should be our guideline. When we are faced with several courses of action, we should study each of them and find out if it is impelled by passions, fear, indolence, and so forth, or whether it will lead to falsity or deception of others— all such actions should be rejected. Again, honest and principled action in which we have no selfish considerations should be our course. No action can be called correct or incorrect in itself; the attitude of the action is the only determining factor. Because all actions have both good and evil results, no action is greater or smaller than another.

A true Karma Yogi, who acts without hankering for the results, will automatically be guided into taking the correct path, as things like passion or anger will not influence him or her. As long as we are acting out of Sattva, whatever course of action we have chosen is the correct one. Only actions guided by Tamas or Rajas are to be avoided. We need to analyze ourselves, rather than the work we do, to ascertain whether we are doing work in the proper way. When something is done in a Sattvic spirit, then we cannot do anything wrong. But when we are doing something with a Rajasic or Tamasic attitude, we are definitely taking a wrong course and need to change.

Hence, Karma Yoga is not without its moral guidelines. But this is different from that of other religions. Hinduism does not have the Ten Commandments of Christianity or the moral guidelines of the Qu'ran. It recognizes that such strict rules would not be applicable for all persons at all times.

Karma Yoga instead shows us how to achieve moral guidelines by changing our personality. It tells us not *what* to do but *how* to do it. It teaches us to always have a Sattvic attitude, free from cruelty, lust, anger, and so on. If we can maintain Sattva, then we will automatically know what action to take in a particular situation. Moral evil in Hinduism is not that which goes against the guidelines of particular texts but that which goes against a Sattvic character and follows Tamas or Rajas. Sattvic people can never do anything evil; they will always do that which is morally right, because they will not be blinded by such things as hunger, anger, and selfishness. They will refrain from evil even when all the forces of society are forcing them to do it. Nor again will they shirk doing anything that needs to be done, even when the entire world is against it. This is the message of Karma Yoga. When we know how take actions in a larger context, we will know how to do individual things also, and be guided into making the correct decision at each step.

If the effort we make cannot influence the results of our work, though, this theory could be seen as demoralizing and leave us with no incentive to work hard. If all actions may have both good and bad results, and even our kindest course of action could harm someone, then there seems no point in doing anything.

Karma Yoga says that, far from demoralizing us, believing in a theory that doesn't look at results is in fact the best way to go about a life of action. Hindu theories are propounded almost like an experimental result, and it is after observation of human attitudes toward work that Karma Yoga propounds its theory. It says, in fact, that it is when we are looking only at the results of the work that we are bound to become demoralized, and work for work's sake is the way to get the best output from ourselves.

Arise and win glory!
Conquer your foes and fulfil your kingship!
They are already killed by me.
Be just my instrument,
The archer at my side!

    —Bhagavad Gita, 11.33

The Bhagavad Gita (The Song of God) is the main spiritual text on Karma Yoga. It is the advice given by Lord Sri Krishna to Arjuna on the battlefield of Kurukshetra in the Mahabharata, and the advice teaches him the correct path to follow at a time of immense turmoil. Arjuna is the main warrior of the Pandavas, and he gears up for battle against the Kaurava army, which is ranged against him. But as he surveys the army, he sees that many of his relatives and friends are against him, and when he realizes that he will have to fight and kill them, he is filled with sorrow and fear and turns away, saying to Krishna, who is acting as his charioteer, that he cannot fight such a battle. The Gita is the poem in which Krishna then gives him advice on how to act, composed in some of the most beautiful Sanskrit verses.

The Gita is set in the battlefield to symbolize the immense moral and emotional trauma that faces us at certain points in life. Arjuna is portrayed to be facing perhaps the greatest moral dilemma that a person could come up against. We are not normally going to come across a challenge like facing our cousins and friends in a war, but even so, the world is our battlefield, and we often have to work against great odds. Many a time we are overcome by doubts of how and whether to act and are racked by pain and frustration. We feel tempted to take the path of least resistance and are not sure what to do. Even in simple everyday decisions, we are confronted by the same essential problems and tensions. The Gita, by showing the path to Arjuna, also acts as our guide at every point of our daily life.

There are many moral questions that haunt Arjuna. What exactly is the method to take to do our work to perfection? How do we maintain our composure when we are faced with several contrary emotional pulls and pressures in doing our work? How do we know what our duty is? Will not doing this duty cause more harm than good?

In reply to this, Krishna sets out the two main principles of Karma Yoga: do your duty without attachment to results, and maintain the quality of Sattva. If we act with detachment, we maintain Sattva, and then we can be sure that whatever duty we perform is correct. We then do our work to perfection and are not diverted by Tamasic or Rajasic emotions.

The Gita also says it is foolish to think that we can determine the results of our actions. They are beyond our control. We have freedom only for work, not for obtaining the results. The Gita then goes on to say that through Karma Yoga, we can also obtain realization and achieve liberation. The teaching here is not how to go to war, but how to fight a war when it falls to our lot. Hence the most abhorrent thing is given as an analogy, a duty that falls to its hero of a war against his own friends and relatives. Krishna shows how even the most hateful duty can be done in accordance with spirituality. When such a thing can be done and the person can still make spiritual progress, every duty that falls to us can lead us onward to spiritual heights. It is not what we do, but how we do it that is important.

That is what Krishna shows Arjuna, that his reaction is not that of Sattva but of Tamas, arising from fear and weakness. If he had only Sattva within himself, he would not have hesitated to fight. Circumstances have prescribed that his duty to his family, to the society, and to justice compels him to fight. He is reluctant, but this reluctance stems from Tamas. Arjuna is making a grave mistake in his attitude to work: he is thinking about the results rather than the work, and it is this that gives rise to Tamas. Arjuna eventually realizes his mistake and becomes Sattvic in nature. He is then able to carry on the fight, which is necessary to establish justice in the land, and fights on to victory.

The Bhagavad Gita is told in a dualistic setting, and it believes in reincarnation. It sets out the law of Karma by which every action of ours will have results at some point, if not in this life, then in a later life. The only way to get freedom from this wheel of Karma is if we act without attachment to results. The results, then, will not react on us. It also describes the paths of Jnana and Bhakti Yoga. (Raja Yoga is not discussed, possibly because it was then a part of the Samkhya Yoga system and had not been adapted into the Vedantic philosophy.)

The Bhagavad Gita shows us the practical path to religion for a person of action. In India, it is the Gita and not the Upanishads that form the practical guide for everyday life, and it is the teachings of this text that are more known and practiced than the esoteric teachings of the Upanishads.

The teachings of Karma Yoga continue to reverberate throughout India, and it had another period of glory during the Indian independence movement, through the leadership of a true Karma Yogi, Mahatma Gandhi. He united the entire country by teaching that the movement was not just a political struggle, but a spiritual one. In his simple words, he taught the essence of Karma Yoga, that the means is important rather than the end.

Mahatma Gandhi showed that the struggle was not just against imperialism, but the individual struggle of each person against their own selves, against the evil in themselves, against their fear, anger, and, most importantly, hatred of the other. The prime duty was to bring out the Sattvic nature in everyone. To maintain this Sattvic nature of the struggle, he developed his own unique forms of political protest through peaceful means, by non-cooperation, hunger strikes, and *satyagraha*. The prime object was not to destroy the enemy but to strengthen oneself, to be invulnerable to the enemy and thus weaken him.

In a country like India, a mere political struggle would not have evoked the raw emotions that Gandhi's spiritual teachings brought about, and it united the whole country irrespective of age, caste, or religion. Through this, India showed once again the hold that spiritualism has on the country, even in modern times.

Karma Yoga must not be seen solely as a path connected to religion. Through the ages and in cultures around the world, the methods of Karma Yoga have been understood and followed by great personalities in their achievements. The need for total absorption in the work itself and the strength that can be derived has been understood by scientists, philosophers, and artists such as musicians, painters, and sculptors from time immemorial. This is not a special secret of Yoga but a universal truth. It is only that in Hinduism, these methods have been employed in spirituality to attain a mystical end.

Karma Yoga is the path for the practical people of action. In the doctrines of the other Yogas, a worldly life is inimical to further knowledge. Those living a worldly life are barred from their spiritual goals. The only way to a spiritual end would be to completely abandon a worldly life. But Karma Yoga shows that the same goals can be attained through a worldly life. It shows us how to tackle the infinite diversions that affect a practical life and how to fulfill our duties and responsibilities in such a way that work leads to realization. The effort is to do perfect work, but not to expect anything from it, and hence not to get attached to it. Once the work is finished, we should be able to rise up from it without thinking about it anymore. When we can live in the world in such a way, our minds become free from the passions and torments that drag us down. Work itself becomes a meditation, and through work, we attain our liberty.

Karma Yoga by itself can lead us to realization, but it also forms the underpinning for those who follow the path of Bhakti, Raja, and Jnana Yoga, for fulfilling their duties. Even Yogis have to do work as long as they are alive, and so Karma Yoga is essential for all. Through Karma Yoga, the other paths—such as Raja and Jnana, which are otherwise barred to householders—become open to all. This path shows us how to use the world, with all its diversions, to find our way to spiritual goals. It is thus immensely strengthening, both for the individual and society, and shows that the life of a practical man is no less spiritually rewarding than that of a philosopher.

~ 13

Jnana Yoga

*"O good looking one, you shine verily like a knower of
Brahman. Who may it be that instructed you?" He confirmed
saying, "Some ones other than human beings. But it is you,
revered sir, who should instruct me to fulfil my wish."*

—**Chandogya Upanishad IV.ix.3**

J nana Yoga is the branch of Yoga that seeks to realize the
absolute truth by meditating on our knowledge of the world.
Jnana Yoga is the chief path to realization described in the
Upanishads. Bhakti and Karma are occasionally mentioned briefly,
but the main purport of the Upanishads is to acquire the mystical experience through *Jnana* (knowledge).

Jnana Yoga is the path followed by the ancient *rishis* of India,
and it is their prophetic insights acquired through this path that
have given rise to Hindu philosophy. Even today, it is the chief
path followed by the ascetics of India. These ascetics are still extant
throughout India, most particularly in the Himalayas, in schools
or "Ashrams," where monks from throughout the country are
drawn and initiated into what is virtually the most demanding
quest for an ultimate answer to life. They are people from all walks
of life, and their caste, language, or social status is immaterial.
They are driven by a burning desire for that which is immortal,
and for this search, they have given up their homes, families,
wealth, and every aspect of a social life. The ancient drama that

once drew the sages of the Upanishads continues to be played out in contemporary India as well, which still has its share of prophets and sages.

Jnana Yoga is traditionally considered to be the hardest and most demanding of the Yoga paths. It is the most unforgiving and demands a complete renunciation of everything that is *maya*. Maya, the enchanting and beguiling nature of the world, is the great enemy, and the Yogis in the Upanishads and other sacred texts of India speak harshly of all temporal attachments. Even qualities like love and kindness are harmful for the Jnana Yogi. They are seen to be equally oppressive and binding. Maya binds us not just by catering to our baser instincts but through our goodness as well. Our love for our dear ones, for our families and children, ties us up as effectively as our baser passions. Things like kindness and compassion for others do the same, as such emotions make us more involved in the world in an effort to help others. This in turn leads us into the arms of maya, and we are diverted from our spiritual quest. Hence Jnana Yogis have to abandon *all* social ties and bindings as they begin their quest.

Such an antisocial teaching is bound to lead to resentment and protests. Indian myths and folklore are often about this tension between the Yogis who have abandoned their all and society's reaction against them. Such an action brings about no benefit to society. It is a lonely quest, and the only benefit the Yogis gain is for they themselves. It was decried as a selfish act, and Yogis were depicted as cold, heartless beings who caused intense suffering to their families and society in response to a sudden selfish whim. On the other hand, traditional Sanskrit dramas often idolized such Yogis, and it was the clinging nature of society that was depicted as detestable.

But all this has little meaning for the Yogis setting out on the quest. The impulse that drives them is the quest for the absolute truth, and this inner compulsion makes abandoning society seem a small sacrifice to find the truth. These are people driven by a desire that few of us can understand, let alone have, and such is the passion that it burns up all other desires that might drive the rest of us.

To the Yogi, all the calls of society are but the traps of maya. They are snares set out to keep us entranced forever in the web of relativity. No matter how strong the calls of society seem, they are still the calls of temporality only. None of our ties are permanent; it is an inevitable fact that we are all going to die. Those who believe in such ties are also deluded, and by remaining with them, we will only become trapped in the same delusion.

Similarly, we cannot make anyone less unhappy through compassion. The mass of suffering and happiness in the world remains constant. If we fulfill someone's material needs, he or she develops new emotional needs that are subtler than before, and the end result is the same. Society has no need for us, and we cannot change anything for those who are trapped in maya. This whole web of maya is like a prison, and unless we can avoid each and every part of its charms, we will remain prisoners, and our desire for the immortal truth will never be fulfilled.

Such calls for sacrifice usually leave most of us unconvinced. It seems like nothing more than Puritanism, and in the modern age, it seems to be a retrograde step. But for the Jnana Yogi, renunciation is the most intelligent thing that can be done. In our everyday life, too, we find that a thinking person will always sacrifice temporary pleasures for a deeper pleasure, even though it may be further away. This is what makes a student concentrate on his books or an office employee work diligently rather than spend time at a bar; it is in expectation of a higher reward for a temporary sacrifice. To the Jnani, foregoing the temporal pleasures of a worldly life is only a preparation for the much greater bliss that he or she is driven to seek.

Normally, when we ask what we seek from life, we would answer with things like a loving family, good friends, money, cars, and so on. But for the Jnanis, the answer is simpler. They would say "happiness." Happiness is what we are all after when we seek these things. People seek wealth because they feel it will bring them happiness; they seek power, love, and more, all in search of this goal.

The Upanishads say that there is a state of the human mind referred to as *ananda*, bliss, or perhaps more accurately, ecstasy, which is the most natural condition of the human mind. It is to regain this state that all our efforts are directed. Because of differentiation into an individual identity, we have fallen away from it. We are struggling all the time to regain this state, but because of our misconceptions, we believe that it is through the attainment of such objects that we will achieve bliss. But the Upanishads say this is not so, as each desire fulfilled will give rise to a thousand others. Instead, it shows us a more direct way to achieve this state, and this is the path of Yoga.

We get different types of pleasure from our worldly desires; the pleasure experienced during sex is different from the pleasure of wealth or love, and so on. All these pleasures are in fact only temporary states of that undifferentiated bliss, which is the root of all these. If we can reach this state, we would get something far higher than the happiness from these worldly objects.

By abandoning temporary desires, we are still ultimately going toward the same end as that of a materialistic person, only this time we are doing it in the right way, the more intelligent way. We are not running after the sparks from the fire but the fire itself. The happiness and bliss that we will achieve at the end of Yoga will be incomparably more intense and fulfilling than anything that we can achieve in a worldly life.

Jnana Yoga is unique in spiritual teachings in that it depends solely on the intellect to bring us to the truth. In the Upanishads, a logical system of reasoning leading to the ultimate truth is built up to support the intellectual conception of Brahman. Jnana Yoga leads us along this path of logic, and by analyzing the world as we see it, we come to the intellectual conception of the Advaitic Brahman.

The aim of Jnana Yoga is to get rid of the delusion in which maya has trapped us. This delusion is called *avidya* in the Upanishads. The delusion consists of the belief that the world around us is real and existent, so that we do not seek out any higher truth beyond it.

Normally we see the world around us as having a solid and real existence and following regular laws of cause and effect with a harmonious flow of time and space. This is the "classical" world of Newtonian physics. But during meditation, the sages discovered that this was not true; the world instead was ill-defined and "fuzzy," and the first impression was incorrect. The sages also discovered simultaneously that there was an absolute beyond it all, and this was the base that gave the world its reality; thus our first view of the world as real is said to be a delusion, or avidya.

By getting rid of the delusion, we come to the knowledge of the truth: that this world is unreal, and only the Brahman is real. This knowledge is called *vidya*. Vidya was characterized by Ramakrishna Paramahamsa as the intellectual realization of this truth. But this intellectual conception is not enough. This is as far as science or logic can lead us.

But Yoga says there is a stage beyond this intellectual knowing of Brahman, a stage of consciousness in which we leave reason and logic behind and come to a direct apprehension of Brahman, and this is the goal of religion. Ramakrishna gave the analogy of a thorn: vidya is a thorn we use to remove the thorn of avidya that is stuck in our flesh. But just as after removing the thorn, we do not need either thorn, after removing avidya, we go beyond intellectual concepts alone and try to achieve the mystical knowledge.

Advaita emphasizes that the knowledge of Brahman as the true reality is simultaneous with the knowledge that the world is unreal. Both are implicit in each other. This comes through arguments and logic in the intellectual conception, but in samadhi, the realization is simultaneous. Once we see Brahman, we do not see the world anymore, as we realize its ill-defined state. So there are basically two ways of *experiencing* existence: first, in our normal state, when we experience the world and our individual identity as real; and second, during samadhi, when we experience Brahman as the sole reality and everything else as unreal.

The analogy given to explain mystical knowledge is that of the rope and the snake. Initially we believe the rope to be the snake, which is like believing this world to be real. But once we have knowledge, we see that in fact it is the rope that is real, and simultaneously we realize that the snake is unreal. Similarly, once we see Brahman, we realize that the world is unreal. Even after coming out of the meditative state, when we may not have direct contact with Brahman, this realization that the world is unreal stays with us, and we are not lured by the world, just as having once known it as a rope we are no longer afraid of the snake.

The Upanishads advise us to first hear, then think, and then practice. Intellectual conviction is necessary for the path to mysticism. This is where the logic and rationality of the Upanishads come to the forefront. For many, faith alone is sufficient for their spiritual efforts. But for many others, something more rigorous— an intellectual conviction—is needed to sustain spirituality. The metaphysical theories of Advaita provide such a basis, as they rely on logic alone without any recourse to doctrines. A rational outlook would provide the strength of mind necessary in our spiritual efforts when doubts arise, as they inevitably must.

> *Taking hold of the bow, the great weapon familiar in the Upanishads, one should fix on it an arrow sharpened by meditation. Drawing the string, o good looking one, hit that fiery target that is imperishable, with the mind absorbed in thought.*
>
> —Mundaka Upanishad 2.2.3

The exercise of Jnana Yoga is directed toward this goal of merger in Brahman. By following the path of meditation prescribed in it, we gradually come to the intellectual conception of Brahman as the ground of both the external and the internal world. As we continue to meditate on this conception, a stage is reached when all reasoning and thinking is stopped, and we come to an immersion in Brahman. This is the state affirmed by the ancient seers of India, and the spiritual goal of Jnana Yoga is to arrive at this stage of mysticism.

Jnana Yoga begins with complete renunciation. The first task of those who seek to attain the immortal truth is to cut themselves off from all attachment to mortal things. The way to do this is in a single stroke. One must suddenly leave everything behind and begin the quest. It is said to be impossible to leave things behind one at a time. Renunciation, of course, is not just distancing oneself physically, but also mentally. Jnana Yogis have become so tired of the enchantments of the world that these have no power to leave any longings in the mind.

There are no definite rules for Jnana Yoga. Once the renunciation is made, the aspirants approach a guru, at which point they are indoctrinated into a particular method of meditation. But the Jnani must always struggle alone; there is nothing that anyone can do to guide them after the initial teachings. The struggle is with their mind, to surpass it, and in this there can be no outside help. The Jnanis meditate alone, in isolated caves in the mountains or forests, coming down only occasionally to replenish their meager stocks. The Himalayan mountains are the famous abode of ascetic schools of India.

The way of meditating in Jnana Yoga is to take up a particular way of reasoning, and to reason along this path until the intellectual conception of Brahman as the only possible answer is firmly fixed. Then one meditates on this conception until a sudden flash of realization comes, when the individual consciousness rises above thinking and reasoning and comes to a stage of direct apprehension and immersion in Brahman, and the aspirants reach their goal.

This flash of realization is what Jnana Yogis spend years preparing for. It is said that to those who had good lives before, this realization can come on quite early. There is a story of a king who had realization as he was getting on a horse, during the moment between putting his foot in the stirrups and climbing on to the saddle. But the majority must struggle for years before this mystical realization dawns on them. All the years of asceticism and meditation are only meant to clear up the mind so it is ready and adequate to receive this knowledge.

Once this stage is realized, the aspirant is freed from all social needs and conventions. When it is realized that all is Brahman, all emotional outputs, such as fear, desire, and disgust, are surpassed. The Yogi is then in a stage of higher conception that cannot be reached by anyone else, and his or her actions or thinking are beyond the understanding of society. The Yogi has reached the stage of absolute freedom.

Yoga can also deteriorate. Constant practice is needed to hold on to the knowledge. As soon as we come out of the meditative state, we are once more assailed by the events of the world, and we fall away from the knowledge. Hence the Jnanis choose to live in isolation and away from all worldly desires in order to perfect their Yoga, so that all their waking moments finally become mystical, and they remain always in contact with the realization.

There are many meditation exercises described in the Upanishads and other texts. All of these are meant to eventually lead to the same goal of realization. One exercise is to meditate on one's own name. By repeating one's name within the mind, we gradually come to see the ideas associated with the name, that it is this identity that binds us to society and all our ties to society are bound up to this name. Our individual consciousness is bound up to our name. Then we gradually realize that our name alone surely cannot encompass us; we are not just the mass of individual consciousness alone but something higher than this, something that is above all this, and this consciousness, this name, restricts us. From this stage, mystical realization can be reached.

Meditation on one's reflection is also done. In this, we see our form as reflected in the mirror consisting of our face and bodies, and by thinking on it, we realize that it is this alone that others see and recognize as us. But this body cannot be the sole representation of ourselves; we are much more than what others see us as. By meditating in this way, we can reach mystical experience.

Similarly, by meditating on a part of one's body, we can reach the same stage. By looking at our hand, we come to think that this hand, this leg, and so on is ours, and that which owns this hand is what we call our individuality. We can never go beyond our body. But we cannot be only the owners of this body; this body is not the sole limit for our true individuality. The body is like a cage for us, and our true individuality is something far beyond this.

By meditating on our birth, we can also see that there appears to be a definite time at which our existence began. Before our birth this "I" did not exist. But we realize that cannot be. There can never be a stage in which we did not exist, and this "I" is only a temporary reflection of our infinite existence.

Similarly, by meditating on our death, we can see that it is impossible that there will come a time when we do not exist. It is only this individual consciousness that will cease to exist, our true "I," the subject of our consciousness, must always continue to exist.

We can also meditate on the infinity of time and space. We can look backward and visualize ourselves going back in time, and realize that no matter how far we go, we can never arrive at the beginning of time, because time has no beginning. Similarly, by going forward, we realize that time is everlasting, and it will never end. This leads us to a timeless sphere, and we can free our individuality from the grip of concepts of time and attain freedom. Similarly, by meditating on the infinity of space, we can attain freedom from concepts of space.

In this way, we can meditate on everything around us and see how it leads to a contradiction, until we come to the realization of Brahman. We can meditate on the room around us and realize that at this particular moment in time and space, we are trapped, as it were, in this room with its objects, in its time and space, and we do not exist outside these limitations. We then realize the impossibility of this as truth, of our true individuality being bound up in this way, and are led to a mystical realization.

Such meditation exercises can be practiced anywhere and at any time. They must be practiced constantly until we are led to a stage in which the world will be seen as a mass of contradictions, and then an absolute truth will dawn beyond it.

The most well-known meditation exercise in the Upanishads is meditating on "neti, neti," "not this, not this." In this, the aspirant denies any conception of Brahman that comes to the mind. We are not capable of conceptualizing the absolute Brahman, and when we try to think of it, we invariably imagine our nearest approach to it, such as the infinite sky, infinite goodness, ether, and so on. The Upanishads say none of this can encompass Brahman. Hence, to each conception that comes to the mind, we say, "Neti, neti." We strike down each conception until the mind does not come to any conceptions anymore, and it is at that moment, when we do not try to limit the Brahman, that we realize it.

Another form of meditation is to constantly say "I am that, I am that." Each time we say this, a momentary impression remains in the mind. Of course, in the ordinary course, the impression is quelled almost at once by a large number of opposing arguments; for example, "if I am that, then why am I not all powerful?" These questions are to be countered with logic such as telling ourselves that these questions themselves arise only in the relative plane, and in the absolute plane, there is only Brahman. By arguing and repeating this as often as we can, gradually the impressions made on the mind become stronger, and finally, the moment of realization is flashed upon.

Another meditation is on fire. In the hymns of the Vedas, all offerings are made to fire, and it is a nature-worshipping ritual. But in the Upanishads, we are asked to see that the offering is not to the fire itself, but to that which is symbolized by fire. At first it is shown that man himself is symbolized by fire, with the eyes its embers, speech the flames, breath the smoke, and so on. The whole universe is shown to be symbolized by fire. Ultimately, we come to realize that all things are one, and the absolute lies beyond it all.

Another such meditation is one in which we are led from the lower or grosser manifestation to the higher or finer. First, we ask whether speech is Brahman. It is shown that it is not speech but the vital force that is finer and lies beyond speech. Then it is shown that the mind lies beyond speech, and so on, through the various stages of existence postulated in the Upanishads, to *akasha* and then *prana*, until, finally, we arrive at Brahman.

Similarly, we merge everything into Brahman. We try to analyze ourselves, whether we are defined by our speech, our mind, and so on; and then we see that it is not such things that define us, but something higher. We then strike down each definition—speech, mind, *prana*, and so on—until we reach Brahman. Then we finally arrive at the conception that we are Brahman itself: "thou art that." This is given in the analogy of bees gathering nectar from different flowers, which becomes honey, in which we cannot distinguish the different nectars. A similar analogy is the rivers merging into the sea.

In all these different ways of meditating, the ultimate goal is the same: to achieve the final state of direct perception of Brahman. Jnana Yoga as defined in the Upanishads is a harsh, lonely path, and it is suitable for only a small number of people who are driven to make the sacrifices called for. But by using Bhakti, we can arrive at a confirmation of the intellectual conception of Jnana Yoga without imposing such sacrifices upon society and ourselves. At the same time, by having Jnana Yoga as the backbone of Bhakti, we will not surrender to empty superstition, nor will we have to lose the strength of reason given by Jnana. By combining Jnana and Bhakti Yoga, we can arrive at a synergistic combination of the strength of both the heart and the mind to arrive at a final, direct realization of the absolute truth.

Advaita in the Modern Context

Hinduism is the oldest of all existing religions. It is not an "invented" religion but an evolved one. It can lay claim to having its roots in the Bronze Age, and even farther beyond to the times of the dawning of our civilization, when humans first began wondering about the world around them and drawing up a philosophy for sustenance. Other religions that developed similarly, of the Greeks, the Egyptians, and the Mesopotamians, have all been subsumed by other religions, mainly by the proselytizing religions spread by determined individuals and groups, such as Christianity and Islam, as well as Buddhism and Jainism. Judaism is a similarly evolved religion, as are the religions of Bushmen, Native Americans, and other, smaller groups. But none of these belief systems have the diversity and strength of the philosophy, logic, and systems of practice that Hinduism has to offer. Taoism in China is also an evolved religion, but it has a later origin.

The political unity of India, *Bharat*, is also almost as ancient. In the Ramayana, Ram sets out on a path of conquest of the entire country. The Mahabharata describes a great civil war that the entire country of Bharat was embroiled in, with kings from as far away as Kamrup, the present Assam, and the southern states joining one camp or the other. From the regions described here from which the different kings came, we see outlined for the first time the area that was considered as belonging to this ancient entity, Bharat. This political organization of the country was recognized since ancient times by civilizations in other parts of the world, and the Greeks and Mesopotamians have always referred to the Indian as a single civilization.

Hinduism is the defining religion of India. It is by far the oldest religion in India, as all other religions came long after. For some centuries Hinduism was supplanted by Buddhism as the most important religion, and most of the country had been converted to a Buddhist way of life. But Hinduism revitalized itself around the first millennium CE to such an extent that Buddhism died out—or, rather, was absorbed so completely that it became a minor religion with only a few isolated groups of followers.

Hinduism may be defined as the system of beliefs based on the Vedas. All Hindu sects ultimately depend on the Vedas. The Vedantic schools of thought, which depend on the Upanishads, are the main stream of Hinduism and continue to be the dominant force. Other schools like *Shaivism* and *Tantricism* do not depend directly on the Vedas, but rather on texts called the *agama* texts, but these again depend on the Vedas. Besides these, other vital texts of the religion like the epics and the Gita depend on the Vedas for their authority. It is this acceptance of the authority of the Vedas that unites the different paths of Hinduism with all their divergences in philosophy, traditions, and practices.

The long course of evolution of the religion, combined with the vibrancy of Indian thought, has given Hinduism a very rich diversity in both schools of thought and systems of practice. In its theory, Hinduism covers the entire gamut of thought, from pure dualism to *Advaita*, including Tantricism, materialism, atheism, and so on. Each such school of thought has numerous tracts and sidetracks; dualism alone has literally hundreds of Ishtas throughout the country, with the relationship between God and worshipper being defined in various ways.

There is also widespread atheism, as in the south, where a political movement based on atheism found widespread support. This does not create any problems in India, and no one would suggest that they are not Hindus.

This arises from a distinctive feature of Hinduism: its spiritual tolerance. A religion has various sides: its philosophical aspect, practices, social aspect, political aspect, and so on. Hinduism has its faults in the social aspect, but on the philosophical side, no other religion and, in fact, very few philosophies, can lay claim to the tolerance espoused within.

"God is one, the wise call it by various names." This is the supreme mantra of tolerance embedded in the Vedas. There is no higher or lesser god in Hinduism; the different gods are but different names of the same supreme power. This is the greatness of Hinduism: that it could say that all streams lead to the same God, and, therefore, all persons are correct by following a spiritual path in their own way. Neither Buddhism nor Islam nor Christianity could ever say this. This belief is still as much a part of modern Hindu life today; even the most ardent Hindu fanatic would still not criticize the God of other religions, no matter how much he attacks their proponents.

Politically, Hinduism has always resisted proselytizing, and this led to violent conflicts with Muslims, as well as more peaceful resistance to Christian missionaries. But Hinduism by itself never favored conversion attempts, and it is to its credit that throughout its long history there were never any Hindu attempts to actively force or convince others to start believing in its gods.

It is in the social sphere that Hinduism showed its disturbing side, with the evil of the caste system throwing a long shadow on the major part of its population. The Bhakti movement emerged as an important tool to lift up those oppressed by the system. In the last two hundred years, especially since independence, democracy has ensured transfer of power to all sections of society and whittled rapidly away at the last vestiges of this system.

The central feature of Hinduism is that it is a mystical religion. The aim of Hinduism is always to seek the union of the material with the divine. There may be differences in philosophy and practices, but the one point that unites all Hindu sects is this goal of mysticism. Hence, Hinduism is always an individualized religion, and its teachings are always for the individual soul seeking realization. There is no collective heaven or some such sphere for all to aspire to. This union of the soul with the absolute is what all the different paths promise as the final fruition for their disciples.

The message of all the great teachers of Hinduism was the same: that all paths lead to the same goal, and therefore it does not matter what path we choose. What is important is that we choose one and practice it until we are led to its culmination. The final message given in Advaita was that even if we follow a dualistic or qualified monistic path, when we reach the final stage, we will be led to the realization of the Advaitic truth *Tat Tvam Asi* (Thou Art That). So no path is false, because they will all ultimately lead to the same end.

Advaita is but one among these streams of Hinduism. It has never been the mainstream, which has always been dualism and qualified monism. Advaita was always considered an esoteric path, difficult to understand and even more difficult to follow. The appeal of Advaita is to the brain and not to the heart. There is in it no supreme power to which we can turn for help. This made it a difficult path for most people to accept, and it mainly remained as a religion of the ascetics in their mountain caves.

Yet for those who desire only the highest truth, the teaching of Advaita remains the beacon. Advaita draws in all those who desire only rationality and clarity, who will not accept anything that they cannot prove for themselves or that is contrary to other knowledge and depends on doctrines, who will not compromise anywhere in their search for the ultimate truth.

The message of Advaita may seem a cold and forbidding one to those who seek comfort from their religion, but for those whose goal is to know the truth, it is the strength of Advaita that draws them forward. For them, all other religions are inadequate, and their goals are only halfway houses. Other paths are at the most mere tools to lead them on to the highest truth, the absolute of the Advaita.

The different paths are not higher or lower. The goal of a true religion is to bring us to a higher truth, a truth that encompasses the qualities that we seek within others and ourselves. It is not that a superior metaphysical theory makes for a superior religion. The basic aim of a religion is to fulfill our spiritual needs, and for that, one does not need philosophy or theories. The great religions in the world have achieved their greatness because, in one way or the other, they have fulfilled this basic spiritual need. A true religion is that which fulfills our yearning for something higher and enables us to reach out for that higher thing.

Each religion fulfils this need in its own way, and because different people have different spiritual needs, each religion has its role. A person has to seek the religion that best fulfills what he or she desires spiritually. No religion can be considered superior or inferior, for they each have their role to play in spirituality.

Advaitism does not lay claim to being the most superior of religions. It claims to be the most rational. But being rational is not the goal of all religions, and Advaitism recognizes this: "We have no quarrel with them." Dualism has as important a role to play as rationalism in religion. Religions that have dualism as their creed are as necessary for the world as those based on rationalism. Similarly, religions based on atheism, such as Buddhism, are necessary, as well as philosophical streams such as qualified monism.

The different needs of individuals make each religion important in its own sphere. Advaita may have the greater logic, but that does not mean it will bring us to the goal of religion any faster. In fact, a simple-minded faith in dualism can often be more efficacious and faster in achieving this supreme goal, depending on the person who is drawn to it. All dualists are not simply credulous persons who do not apply logic in their thinking. Some of the greatest scientists and thinkers have been thorough-going dualists. They have found in their religion the deep faith that fulfills a person's spiritual needs and, in the light of which, all reason and logic seems dry and bare.

The differences in different religions need to be there because they appeal to different mindsets. Each must have the freedom to accept the path that is most suitable for him or her. The difference is both in the philosophy and in the practice. Even when the metaphysical beliefs are more or less the same, there are differences in cultural values; within dualism, for example, there are Christian, Islamic, and Hindu beliefs, and each may accept the path that most appeals to his or her higher feelings. Within the same religion again, there are usually many different practice systems, such as those of reason, love, and ritualism, so in the same religion, a person can find the path that is most suitable to him or her.

There is no question of superiority of religions; instead we must only consider which religion is best suited to us. Christianity is the religion of love, and its central tenets are all built around this precept; Islam again is the religion of faith, and this is its guiding principle. These are all vital fundamentals of religion from which no person can afford to cut him or herself away.

Even as each religion evolved to fulfill its own niche in spirituality, there have always been attempts to combine different streams of thought. Since the beginning, there have been various Bhakti saints who have combined Advaita with Bhakti and shown that Bhakti is not alien to the power of the Advaitic metaphysics. Teachers like Sankardeva in Assam, Tulsidas, and Chaitanya have always preached the highest logic for those who desired this strength. At the beginning of the nineteenth century CE, there arose another teacher in Bengal, Ramakrishna Paramahamsa, who saw the innate richness of both these streams and made them both accessible. His disciple, Swami Vivekananda, took his ideals forward and related Advaita to modern philosophy and science and thus showed its suitability for the present age.

The genius of Ramkrishna Paramahamsa lay in the combination of Advaita with all the systems of Yoga: Jnana, Raja, and Karma, but especially Bhakti. Thus he spoke of practicing, and he himself practiced Hinduism, Christianity, and Islam. He also practiced all the different forms of Yoga. He declared that they all led to the same goal. By combining Advaita with Bhakti, he gave them both the power that each was lacking on its own. Advaita became richer and stronger with the infusion of the love and emotional strength of Bhakti. Bhakti, in turn, became strengthened by the rigor of Advaitic rationalism.

Ramkrishna Paramahamsa showed that Brahman, viewed from the relative viewpoint, could only be seen as a *Saguna* Brahman, a Brahman with qualities. It is only in the highest meditative state that we can see Brahman free from all qualities as *Nirguna* Brahman. Hence all the gods of Hinduism are forms of this Saguna Brahman and do not contradict Advaitism. Hence Bhakti is not just a temporary tool of the Advaitist but very much a part of his struggle and the essence of his strength. It is difficult for a rational person to accept completely the dualistic or qualified monistic gods. But through Advaita, he or she can access the immense strength and love of Bhakti and progress on his spiritual quest.

This teaching was carried on further by his extraordinary disciple, Swami Vivekananda. He applied the language and theory of modern science to the Advaitic principles, and showed how its teachings were so consistent with science. Thus their teachings have shown Advaita in a new light. It is no longer just an esoteric philosophy. Instead its teachings are all the more relevant in the light of modern scientific advance, and Advaita was recast as the religion that can most support the spiritual needs of the present age.

The teaching of Advaita is not confined to a particular religion. This universal truth has been taught and experienced by teachers in all religions. Hinduism has only systematized it and provided the formal framework for its philosophy, whereas in other religions, it remained more or less a doctrinal statement of a few teachers.

In Hinduism we find this idea expressed in bold and strong language and set out on a base of logic and rationality. Its practices were also standardized and argued out comprehensively. The logic of Advaita has never been disputed in Hinduism; what is often disputed is its interpretation of the Vedantic sutras. The chief conflict that others had with it is that it rules out the authority of a supreme loving god above us, and this is what most people in a religion seek.

Yet the force of a unified, absolute principle behind all existence has struck savants throughout the world. The religious literature of mystics in all religions and cultures often contain references to this idea. It might be expressed in allegorical language, and more often than not, those who expressed this absolute reductionism had to face ridicule even from other mystics. Yet it was always there.

The purity of a philosophy that does not depend on any doctrines but instead on an uncompromising search for truth alone is bound to attract minds from all religions. But even people belonging to other religions can accept this without leaving behind their own religion. Christians and Muslims who follow Advaitism may have to leave behind some of the more orthodox tenets of their religion, but various mystics in both religions have left these behind countless times before. They have already crafted a religion built around Jesus and Allah but with qualified monism, and even sometimes monism, as its metaphysics. It cannot be said that only the orthodox interpretation of a religion is the correct one; these mystics have as much a base as the Orthodox Church or mullahs.

Thus followers of these religions who come to believe in Advaitic metaphysics do not need to feel that they are accepting something alien to their religion. This was an important idea often expressed by Swami Vivekananda. Christians need not give up on Christianity to follow Advaitism, because they only need to understand the message of Christ in the light of Advaita. Similarly, Muslims only need to re-appreciate the message of their own religious teachers in the light of Advaita to experience spirituality.

But where Hinduism can be most helpful is in the sphere of practice, in the forge toward mystical experience. Because in Hinduism mysticism has always been the goal of spirituality, many different systems of practice have grown to achieve mysticism. Accordingly, four main paths of Yoga have been developed. This is where Hinduism can help others: by giving them an appropriate method of practice. Disciples can select the method that they find the most appropriate for themselves. In other religions, such detailed and varied methods are not taught, and the mystical experience happens more or less by accident and to individual teachers.

It is only Buddhism that stands in total contrast to Advaitism. One can be both an Advaitist and a Christian or a Muslim, but one cannot be both a Buddhist and an Advaitist. The two religions, developed on the same soil, stand fundamentally opposed to each other in their principles. Yet both are remarkably similar in various ways. Both are the result of an uncompromising search for the truth, and in both we find the message of supreme strength for the individual and no other power. Both religions do not recognize God and only seek the truth.

In fact, we ourselves are this truth. The truth is not to be found in temples, books, rituals, or supplication; the truth is to be sought inside us. There is none to seek favors from or to kneel down to. Both are immensely strengthening religions, because in both we are right at this moment the truth itself. We do not have to change anything, we only need to realize this and cut out the falsehood, and we will see ourselves as we really are. But there is an irreconcilable polarity in the way the truth is defined by each, and perhaps only the progress of human knowledge shall one day show us which philosophy is more appropriate to describe reality.

The advances in our knowledge and understanding during these two hundred years have wrought a paradigm shift in human history. The base of human knowledge, on which most religions developed, has changed almost completely. Few religions or philosophies can now claim to conform to present science. This can be met in only two ways, either by rejecting science or by rejecting religion.

We find this happening everywhere. But Advaita shows us a way in which we can reconcile the call of spirituality coming from our souls with our need for truth. Advaita remains the only religious path that concurs with modern science. Not only that, the progress in science is in fact bringing our definition of the world increasingly closer to that of the ancient Advaitists. Advaita has emerged as a vital counterpart on the spiritual side to the progress of scientific knowledge of the present age. Advaita has become even stronger with our increasing understanding of the world around us, and its call of "awake, arise and stop not 'til the goal is reached" resounds with ever-greater vigor.

7

Sources

Chapter 6

Page 105: "That which is beyond the eye is the same as that which is beyond the sun."—Chandogya Upanishad, I.vii.5

Page 107: "By his light all this shines."—Mundaka Upanishad, II.ii.10

Page 108: "Through his luster all these are variously illumined."—Chandogya Upanishad, II.ii.15

Page 115: "that from which all words turn back."—Taittiriya Upanishad, II.iv.1

Page 131: "This is all. Beyond this there is nothing."—Prasna Upanishad, VI.vii

Page 133: "Then, this one who is fully serene, rising up from this body and reaching the highest light, remains established in his true nature. This is the Self. This is Immortal. This is Brahman. Truth is the name of this Brahman who is such."—Chandogya Upanishad, VII.iii.4

Page 134: "'I am the juice of this tree,' 'I am the juice of that tree,' so also, O good looking one, all these creatures, after merging into existence, do not understand this."—Chandogya Upanishad, VI.ix.2

"As they do not realize there, 'I am this river,' 'I am that river,' in this very way indeed."—Chandogya Upanishad, VI.x.2

The Brahma sutras say, "(When the Jiva) has attained (the highest light) there is manifestation (of its real nature)."—Brahma Sutras 4.4.1

"(The Jiva in the state of liberation exists) as inseparable (from Brahman)." —Brahma Sutras 4.4.4

"Being but Brahman, he is merged into Brahman."—Brihadaranyaka Upanishad IV.iv.6

"Just as the lifeless slough of a snake lies in the anthill, so does this body lie. Then the Self becomes disembodied and immortal, becomes the Prana, becomes the Brahman."—Brihadaranyaka Upanishad,IV.iv.7

Page 166: "Ahm Brahmasvi—I am Brahman."—Brihadaranyaka Upanishad I.iv.10

Page 138: "The Self should be realized—should be heard of, reflected on and meditated upon."—Brihadaranyaka Upanishad,II.iv.5

Chapter 8

Page 212: "Of this world it cannot be said that it exists, not exists, both exists and not exists and neither exists nor not exists"

This is a common Buddhist formula expressed in several texts, for example:

"It is not expressed if the Buddha after his death exists,

Or does not exist, or both, or neither."—Mulamadhyamakakarika of Nagarjuna, 25.17

Page 236: "The truth is one, the wise call it by various names."— Rig Veda 1.164.46c

". . . which arouses respect . . ."—Patanjali Yoga Sutras: Concentration:39

Chapter 9

Page 262: "What is that knowledge, by knowing which, all this can be known?"—Mundaka Upanishad, I.i.3

Chapter 10

Page 280: "I am That, I am That."—The mantra of "Hamso, soham" in the Mahavakya Upanishad.

Selected Bibliography

Ackerman, Robert. *Theories of Knowledge: A Critical Introduction*. New Delhi: Tata McGraw-Hill, 1965.

Chetia, Bepin. *Advaitavada in Sankardeva's Theology*. Kolkata: Dr. Padmeswar Gogoi Studies, 1999.

Danino, Michael, and Sujata Nair. *The Invasion That Never Was*. Mysore: Mira Aditi, 1996.

Frawley, David. *The Myth of The Aryan Invasion of India*. New Delhi: Voice of India, 1994.

Gandhi, M. K. *An Autobiography: Or, the Story of My Experiments with Truth*. Ahmedabad: Navajivan Publishing House, 1927.

Gupta, Mahendranath and Swami Nikhilananda, trans. *The Gospel Of Sri Ramakrishna, Vol. I*. Kolkata: Sri Ramakrishna Math, 1985.

——. *The Gospel Of Sri Ramakrishna, Vol. II*; Kolkata: Sri Ramakrishna Math, 1985.

Hawking, Stephen. *A Brief History of Time*. New York: Bantam Books. 1998.

Heil, John. *Philosophy of Mind, A Contemporary Introduction*. New Delhi: Routledge, 2003.

Kempis, Thomas à. *The Imitation of Christ*. Mineola, NY: Dover Publications, 2003.

Miller, Barbara Stoler, trans. *The Bhagavad Gita: Krishna's Counsel in Time of War*. New York: Bantam Classics, 1986.

Miller, Barbara Stoler. *The Gitagovinda of Jayadeva*. Delhi: Motilal Banarsidass, 1992.

Monks of the Ramakrishna Order. *Meditation*. Kolkata: Sri Ramakrishna, 1979.

Mukherjee, Dilip Kumar. *Chaitanya*. Delhi: National Book Trust, 1970.

Nagendra, H. R. *The Art and Science of Pranayama*. Kolkata: Vivekanandna Kendra, 1993.

Nehru, Jawaharlal. *The Discovery of India*. Delhi: Oxford University Press, 1999.

——. *Glimpses of World History*. Delhi: Oxford University Press, 1989.

Neog, Maheswar. *Sankardeva*. Delhi: National Book Trust, 1967.

Radhakrishnan, S. *Indian Philosophy Vols. I and II*. New Delhi: Oxford University Press, 1997.

Rolland, Romain and E.F. Malcolm-Smith, trans. *The Life of Ramakrishna*. Kolkata: Advaita Ashrama, 1986.

——.*The Life of Vivekananda and the Universal Gospel*. Kolkata: Advaita Ashrama, 1988.

Singh, Devendra. *Tulsidas*. Delhi: National Book Trust, 1971.

Sister Nivedita. *The Master As I Saw Him*. Kolkata: Udbodhan Office, 1962.

Swami Gambhirananda, trans. *Chandogya Upanishad*. Commentary by Sri Shankaracharya. Kolkata: Advaita Ashrama, 1992

——. *Eight Upanishads Vol. I*: Kolkata: Advaita Ashrama, 1991.

——. *Eight Upanishads Vol. II*: Kolkata: Advaita Ashrama, 1992.

——. *Mandukya Upanishad*. Commentary by Sri Shankaracharya); Kolkata: Advaita Ashrama, 1979.

Swami Madhavananda, trans. *Brihadaranyaka Upanishad*, Commentary by Sri Shankaracharya. Kolkata: Advaita Ashrama, 1993.

——. *Mimamsa Paribhasa of Krsna Yajvan*. Kolkata: Advaita Ashrama, 1996.

——. *Vairagya Satakam of Bhartrihari*. Kolkata: Advaita Ashrama, 1981.

——. *Vivekasudamani by Sri Shankaracharya*. Kolkata: Advaita Ashrama, 1992.

Swami Vireswarananda. *The Brahma Sutras*. Commentary by Sri Shankaracharya. Kolkata: Advaita Ashrama, 1993.

—— and Swami Adidevananda. *The Brahma Sutras (according to Sri Bhasya of Sri Ramanuja)*, Kolkata: Advaita Ashrama, 1996.

Swami Vivekananda. *Raja Yoga: Or, Conquering the Internal Nature*. Kolkata: Advaita Ashrama, 1990.

Swami Virupakshananda, trans. *Samkhya Karika of Isvara Krsna*. Kolkata: Vedanta Press, 1995.

The Complete Works of Swami Vivekananda, Vols. I to VIII. Kolkata: Advaita Ashrama, 1989.

The Life of Swami Vivekananda by His Eastern and Western Disciples, Vols. I & II. Kolkata: Advaita Ashrama, 1989.

About the Author

PALASH JYOTI MAZUMDAR lives with his family in the city of Guwahati, Assam, India, where he practices medicine. Born in 1970, his ancestors came from the temple town of Hajo, where they have long been associated with the ancient temple of Hayagrib Madhob. Mazumdar's writing is influenced by the many streams of spiritual thought that permeate Indian society, particularly those of Assam; the teachings of Ramakrishna Paramahamsa and Swami Vivekananda have also influenced his outlook.